One Drop of Water

Jason Tyler McLean

Copyright © 2021 Jason Tyler McLean

All rights reserved.

ISBN:

DEDICATION

I dedicate this book to anyone who is fighting a silent battle within themselves. For all the people that feel lost or alone that have not found their way home. For those who have been hurt, torn, or broken by the experiences of their life and are struggling to see a way out. This book is dedicated for any induvial that wants to make positive changes in the state of their mental health in hopes of living an improved way of life. Lastly, this book is dedicated to those who live in denial, fear or perhaps are not educated in the subject matter of mental health and mental illness. I hope these words reach you all.

A special thank you to all those who have helped me along the way. You mean more to me than you will ever know.

CONTENTS

INTRODUCTION

THE MONSTER IN THE SHADOWS

The scariest monsters are the ones that lurk within our souls.
Edgar Allen Poe

Among us there is a monster lurking in the shadows. A silent and savage abnormality. It conceals itself inside every shadow of fear, pain, loss, loneliness, sickness, abuse, trauma, and tragedy. Wherever there is light, there is a shadow for it to hide in. This shadow monster is calm and cunning. Molding and morphing its shape to whatever it must in order to get closer to its prey. It can be as big as our entire world yet can be as small as one tiny fragment of a moment. Age, gender, race or where or how you live mean nothing to it, in its ever-consuming hunger for human life. All that matters to it is that its victims are alive. It will silently ambush and attack anyone it can, with the purpose to infest and infect as many lives as possible. Just like a spider waiting motionlessly in its web for its prey to become entangled in its intricately designed trap. And just like that spider, when that perfect moment arises the shadow monster swiftly attacks its prey injecting its venom into it. This venom is paralyzing for all bitten, but it can affect people differently throughout any stages of their lives. Some will slowly be infected over the course of their lifetime, the venom appearing, disappearing, and then reappearing causing the feeling that life is becoming meaningless and is slowly fading away from them as they lose everything that once made them happy. Others will be hit hard by the paralyzing venom instantly and stand still their entire lives never moving forward again, entangled in the webs of darkness in the corners of the cellars in their minds. Some will think they will never be bitten and therefore are free of the shadow monster's relentless and ravenous appetite. Then suddenly, tragedy or trauma strikes in their life and the shadow monster moves in with lightning-fast precision. Quickly biting into them, its fangs deliver venom so strong that it holds them hostage in that moment for the rest of their living years, trapping them with all the pain and suffering of it, until they die a slow and miserable death.

Once the monster is inside your mind it will slowly start to convince you that you are worthless and that your life has no meaning or purpose. It will devour your creativity and dreams. Pushing an overemphasis on your loneliness, guilt, shame, insecurities, and your weaknesses. It will use your own mind against you and stretch the pain further and further and hold you in it longer every time. Distorting your perception of yourself. Separating you from reality. It will tell you to quit, to give up, not to believe in yourself, that there is no hope and if it has its way ultimately with you... It will tell you to end your life.

The monster in the shadows is Mental Illness and its venom is Depression, Anxiety Disorders, Postpartum Stress Disorder, Bipolar, PTST, Borderline Personality Disorder, Schizophrenia, Body Dysmorphic Disorders, Addiction and Substance Abuse, ADHD, and so many more neurological and mental disorders within its composition. That is why the venom is so precariously threatening because it is in a constant state of adaptation and being composed of so many diversified variables, meaning different illnesses, diseases, and disorders from minor to lethal in the affliction to the mind and potentially the body of every individual it infects. But it does not stop there. Mental Illness can spread from person to person. Genetically, Biologically, Developmentally and Environmentally. It has become a true worldwide Pandemic that receives little media attention and certainly has no psychological propaganda being blasted daily by social media showcasing the reality of its impact on human life.

What is Mental Illness? A generalized term for a recognized, medically diagnosable illness or disease that results in the significant impairment of an individual's cognitive, affective, and relational abilities. Mental Illness can make work, relationships, and other demands extremely difficult. An occasional or long-lasting condition that alters thinking, moods, and behaviors like Depression for an example. As well as having dramatic implications on the state of mental health of the individual. Mental health is the state of well-being of the mind through how we think, feel, and behave. How we handle stress and cope with life's adversity. Similar in elementary comparison to the state of our physical health. Generally speaking, the healthier we are, the better we feel.

The terms Mental Health and Mental Illness are frequently and improperly used reciprocally as the same subject. They are not the same thing. The difference being that everyone always has a level of Mental health be it optimal or poor, just like physical health. Whereas not everyone has a Mental Illness, just like physical illness does not affect everyone at the same time. There can be an overlap of symptoms. A constant poor state of mental health can have psychosocial impairments accompanied with severe distress like depression. In fact, the state of poor mental health is more prevalent than depression, commonly.

The diagnosis of a mental illness or mental disorder can be somewhat controversial and confounding. In my years of seeing a plentiful number of different therapists, phycologists, and psychiatrists, that started way back in my childhood, I have been diagnosed or perhaps misdiagnosed or been suggested with several mental illnesses and disorders. I would like to share all the titles which were bestowed upon me and at what age group. Please allow me to introduce myself. (Drum roll please)

- Clinical depression- teenager, adult
- ADHD (attention-deficit/hyperactivity disorder)-child (ADD), teenager, adult
- Borderline Personality Disorder- teenager, adult
- Bi-polar disorder (manic depression)- teenager
- OCD (obsessive compulsive disorder)- adult
- ARND (alcohol related neurological disorder)- teenager
- Post-Traumatic Stress Disorder- adult
- Narcissistic Personality Disorder- adult
- Body Dysmorphia- adult
- Autism Spectrum Disorder- adult
- Psychopath-child
- Sociopath- teenager
- Substance Abuse Disorder-adult

Quite an impressive roll call. That is the tricky nature of Mental illness and the various disorders under the same umbrella. Many of the above-mentioned mental illnesses and disorders share a complex range of disabilities in neurodevelopment and behavior, adaptive skills, and self-regulation. As well as tremendous difficulty with impulse control, judgment, managing emotions, memory, and attention. Learning and cognitive challenges surface with many of the above as well. During my childhood and teenage years many of the diagnoses were in their infancy stage as it was back in the eighties. A great deal of research and investigation has changed over the last few decades, as more information has been revealed through documented case studies, surveys, testing, analysis, as well as overall improvements in science specifically dedicated to mental health.

The varying and conflicting opinions supplied by the various experts on what was "wrong with me" made the whole process extremely emotionally grueling for my family and myself growing up. As I continued to search for answers over the span of the next twenty years in my adulthood, it had become apparent that the people that I met with to discuss the state of my mental health had differing viewpoints on the nature of my condition. Dissimilar frames of reference. Uncertainty camouflaged in over confidence in ability it would seem like to me. In their defense, I will say that as I became more adept in the articulation of my experiences and behaviors, the diagnosis process became more streamlined, efficient, and definitive later in my adult years.

The main groups of mental disorders are:

- Mood disorders (such as depression, bi-polar disorder)
- Anxiety disorders (such as OCD, social anxiety disorder)
- Behavioral disorders (such as ADHD)
- Personality disorders (such as borderline personality disorder, narcissistic personality disorder)
- Psychotic disorders (such as schizophrenia)
- Eating disorders (such as anorexia, bulimia nervosa)
- Substance abuse disorder (drug addiction-pharmaceutical and illegal drugs)
- Alcohol use disorder (alcohol abuse, alcohol dependence)
- Trauma related disorders (such as post-traumatic stress disorder)

The World Health Organization's website states that one in four people in the world will be affected by a mental or neurological disorder in their lives. Approximately 800 million people are currently living with a mental illness/disorder every year. If substance use disorders the number jumps close to one billion people. Depression and anxiety disorders count for almost six hundred million cases globally. Nearly one million people die each year from suicide. That is a person taking their life every forty seconds. These statistics from The World Health Organization's website are outdated and from 2017. As it seemed to be very complicated and confusing to find any current or accurate statistics online. It is estimated that these numbers will only continue to dramatically increase with the conflicted conditions of the world today. These people are gone forever leaving everyone around them to suffer life altering pain. I was almost one of those people. People that commit suicide could be anybody, people like your mother, your father, your children, your sister, your brother, your lover, your best friend, your relative, the kid at the grocery store that always smiled when they spoke to you, your co-worker, young girls and boys, people that had never had a chance due to severe abuse and trauma, the broken hearted, the broken minded, that person you ignored and didn't call back when they needed your help or that person you should have checked in on one more time, the people who tried to get help but were mocked or told to get over it because they are just sad, the people that lost their loved ones, the ones with sickness and disease, and all the people that truly believed there was undeniably no other way out. For every suicide death there are twenty attempts, making that around twenty-five million suicide attempts per year worldwide. People with Depression and similar psychiatric conditions account for ninety percent of all deaths by suicide. Suicide is the leading cause of death in people aged fourteen to twenty-six years old globally. People with severe Mental Disorders on average tend to die earlier than the general population. This is referred to as premature mortality. There is a ten-to-twenty-five-year life expectancy reduction in patients with severe mental disorders. Most of these deaths are due to chronic physical medical conditions such as cardiovascular diseases including coronary heart disease, atherosclerosis, hypertension, and stroke, as well as respiratory and infectious diseases, diabetes, and suicide according to The World Health Organization's website.

The Our World in Health website states as follows: Mental Health Disorders remain widely under-reported. This is true across all countries, but particularly at lower incomes where data is scarcer, and there is less attention to treatment for mental health disorders.

According to the Public Health Agency of Canada, the national number is just over four thousand deaths by suicide on average per year. That equates to eleven people every day that take their life. That is one person killing themselves every two hours and eighteen minutes in Canada, making it the ninth leading cause of death. Seventy five percent of those deaths are by males. I firmly believe that these numbers are underestimated by miscalculations nationally and globally since many drugs and alcohol related suicide overdose deaths are not recorded as suicides. As well many families will ask the coroners not to put suicide as the cause of death out of shame and how it may look upon them to others. Then there are the people that took their lives that had nothing or without family from the streets, that may have been falsely counted as Covid deaths instead of the true cause of death, which contributes to this miscalculation sadly as well.

Teens are more depressed than ever. Pressures from school, online shaming and bullying, the completely unrealistic standards of beauty portrayed through social media "influencers", "models" and plastic sell out celebrities. Present day parents are addicted to more pharmaceutical drugs, alcohol and so many other substances more than ever before. There are also more drugs available every day on the streets and in the pharmacies. With most people addicted to their phones and the social media apps on them. These combined have skyrocketed the rate of death by suicide with teenagers. Sadly, many depressed teens have not been diagnosed or treated for depression.

LGBTQ+ youth are especially vulnerable to mental health concerns and face increased risk of substance abuse and suicide. LGBTQ+ youth are fourteen times the risk of suicide then straight cisgender youth. Stigma, discrimination, rejection, violence, trauma, bullying, prejudice put these youth at an alarmingly higher risk according to the519.org website.

The Canadian Mental Health Association website states that it estimated that twenty percent of Canadian youth are affected by a mental illness or disorder. The total number of twelve-to-nineteen-year-olds in Canada at risk of developing depression is a staggering three point two million. Canada's youth suicide rate is the third highest in the industrialized world. In Canada only one in five children who need mental health services receive them. That needs to change. Teens that thinking about suicide might do as follows:

- Talk about suicide or death
- Hint that they may not be around for much longer
- Isolate from family and friends
- Talk about feeling guilty and feeling hopeless
- Write songs, poems or letters about heartbreak, separation, and death
- Begin giving away treasured possessions to friends and siblings
- Engage in high-risk behaviors like running away or substance abuse

- Have changes in sleeping and eating habits
- Lose the desire to go to school, sports, and favorite activities
- Have difficulty concentrating, paying attention, or thinking rationally

The CMHA website also states that one in five Canadians in any given year will be affected with a mental illness or mental health problem. By the age of forty, about fifty percent of the population will have had a mental illness. Major depression and anxiety disorders combine for eleven percent of the population. Eating disorders affect approximately one million Canadians. They impact women at a rate ten times that of men and have the highest mortality rate among mental illnesses. Substance use disorders affect approximately six percent of Canadians. Four thousand and twelve Canadians died by suicide in 2019. In Canada, suicide disproportionately impacts Indigenous peoples; the rates of suicide among First nations are three times higher than among non-Indigenous Canadians, and nine times higher among Inuit.

As alarming as the statistics are, what is equally as devastating is that studies show that up to sixty percent of people living with a Mental Illness will never get properly diagnosed or receive appropriate treatment. This heartbreaking fact is caused by the massive roadblock of stigmatization and dogma surrounding Mental Illness. The barriers of judgement and criticism by family, friends, coworkers, and society are like bricks stacked up making walls that are often unclimbable for those affected. Lack of proper public resources combined with way too long extended wait times and the fear of disclosing mental health/illness to unsupportive/uneducated minds make up the mortar that solidifies the impenetrability of these walls for many who seek care. This stigma leads to discrimination against those who have Mental Illness and all too often, sadly the harshest judgments come from the ones that should be from we look to for support. The negative stereotyping comes from a lack of understanding and fear. Inaccurate and misleading media representations are at the nucleus of this issue. The word "mental" has so many negative connotations linked to it. Mental hospital, mental patient, mental problems etc... Mental Illness is a brain that is compromised or not functioning in a neurotypical way. Chemical imbalances for an example can be a root of a Mental illness or disorder. However, those affected by this are often looked down upon. Yet if someone had a tumor in their brain the reception to that would be far more sympathetic.

Take a minute and imagine how that feels. Imagine that your life has been a constant struggle to do the very basics of a "normal life", but you have done everything in your power to carry on. You are aware of the impact that your symptoms have had on you over your life and are dealing with the ups and downs that brings. You have now run into a series of trauma and tragedy. You desperately need help. You want to seek care. Your symptoms are getting worse by the day. You have worked and contributed to a health plan on every paycheck for years with your employer. But due to the increased physiological stress of the fact that you already live with the difficulties personally of a Mental Illness and now must face the opinions of others to ask if you can take a short-term leave of absence to get some help becomes terrifying. One day you muster up all the courage that you have and present your case to the person at your workplace that oversees your benefit program and then they tell you that it is not going to happen, that you will not be granted a leave due to depression. They tell you that you are probably just sad and that you will get over it, eventually. They say that maybe try working harder and that will keep you busy. You agree with them publicly, but inside you are broken. Imagine how that feels as you walk back to your desk and must not only swallow up the feelings of being let down, but also admitting that you needed help and that that need was not met by the resource provided for you that you pay for. Now you are not sure how you will make it. Your distress level blasts off like a rocket uncontrollably into the sky which only makes your symptoms worsen. Imagine how discouraging that would be.

That was my experience at a previous place of employment. I am positive that many people can relate to this. Even more so, there are so many more people that will never bother to make the attempt to get help. They remain voiceless. Unheard. Crippled by the fear of harsh judgement and scrutiny. I often wonder if I would have killed myself that day if the viewpoint of the severity of Mental Illness might have changed. Sadly, oftentimes it takes tragedy to open a closed mind when it has become too late to help someone. Being sad is not a Mental Illness. Depression is.

Learning more about Mental Illness and mental health is an imperative step in disabling stigma, deterring prejudice and discrimination while synchronously encouraging early identification and effective treatment promoting recovery. That is on every person to become a part of.

Mental health Disorders/Mental Illness are very complex and take on so many different forms. Signs and symptoms can vary, depending on the disorder, circumstances, and personal history.

Often when we think of someone with Mental Illness which is a brain illness or disorder, we often think of the extremes like crazy people we see in the streets, people breaking down and being put in a psych ward, we think that it would never happen to us. As well, the common perception about depression and anxiety disorders are that people are looking for attention, to be felt sorry for, that they are lazy, have no drive and they should just get over it. When a person is having trouble controlling their behavior and reacts differently to a situation than the common mold, we say that person is mental, again referring to them as crazy. I believe some of the dogma of Mental Illness originated here with that reference in its title.

These brain illnesses, disorders and neuro diseases can be just as devastating as cancer, crippling as severe Rheumatoid arthritis, and debilitating just like lupus and other autoimmune diseases. Yet, common misjudgment and discrimination against those with a mental disorder still commonly exists. The energy source of the flood is ignorance destroying whatever or whoever is in its path. The devastation left behind is the result of the gravity of stigmatization. The questions I ask are as follows:

Do you honestly believe that anyone with mental illness or behavioral disorders wanted to be born with chemical imbalances or brain malfunction that would present an entire theme park where many of the rides and exhibits were broken down but still being used as though they were not? Facing challenges in their everyday life for as long as they lived? Some are so severe that it would handicap their brain function and formation. Do you think that many of these individuals asked for the traumatic childhood events that would cause destruction and incapability of their growing brain to function properly? Do you think that these kids asked for their lives to be so arrestingly affected by trauma and abuse that not only is their trust shattered for life and will be replaced with shame, guilt, fear, and pain but so is the likelihood of their brain ever coming close to developing to its full potential? What about those whose lives are slowly and painfully taken away with long term sickness? The trauma incurred by that could set up for many brain disorders to take root inside their minds. Millions of those kids have now grown up with mental illness. Many people still live-in denial. Others, too afraid to make a stand. On the positive side of things, there are also a great many that have succeeded in finding their way. And many more will.

As I did more and more research online regarding the state of mental illness worldwide, I came across so many websites from all over the world. In fact, I read many articles from even worldwide organizations for mental health and depression. Statistics and metrics of mental illness globally are inadequately stated. What's more, many of these websites included the topic of the burden of mental illness. Many countries' websites dedicated to mental illness and depression have similar articles relating to the burden of mental illness economically and statistically. I found it very disturbing, in fact I took it somewhat personally. Was I to think that I'm a burden on society because I was born with neurological damage and my brain doesn't produce chemicals the same as everybody else's brain and that I was exposed to severe trauma and abuse throughout my childhood, my early teen years, into my adult life? Even though I have worked since I was fifteen years old and paid into the system for decades and yet I have never received a dime regarding any compensation for living with mental illness. And if I'm costing the system and contributing to an economic burden, I had to ask myself why?

I dug a little deeper into this topic. and what I found was mind blowing as I read more and more statistics from around the world. I came across startling numbers for the treatment and resources available for individuals with a mental illness, specifically depression and anxiety. As I explored the economics of the so-called burden, I began to come up with a very common theme from around the entire world. The available treatment for someone with a mental illness and resources, education is the true failure of this worldwide pandemic. With many countries unable to properly diagnose, treat and rehabilitate individuals with depression so that they can become more efficient within their own life, become productive in the workforce contributing to the economy and perhaps alluring the cost of medication spent to the government's medical plans. What I gathered was the true burden on society from mental illness is the lack of proper treatment, funding, resources, and education, perhaps the dogma and stigma associated with mental illness could be contributing factors to why there is such low numbers of documented cases of such low numbers of people willing to get properly diagnosed due to fear of harsh judgment criticism based on society's standards. According to The World Health Organization, the global average for funding for "mental health" from countries' health budget plans hovered around a deplorable 3%. If that is not the most disturbing example of lack of understanding the dominating force in which Mental illness is in our world, I don't know what else is. These statistics are the most parsimonious insult illustrated by the world's health official's ignorance. It doesn't hail from lack of material and resources at their fingertips, it comes from lack of understanding current trends in neurology, psychology and turning a blind eye to a true pandemic that is running rampant in our world today. It appears to me that these governments like to showcase their awareness of mental illness and mental health issues on the main stage for everybody's viewing pleasure and boast proclamations but do nothing proactive about it. Having a National Mental Health Awareness Month in May, here in Canada is amazing and has significantly raised awareness. However, given the current metrics of the ever-increasing numbers of those affected by mental illness and disorders in our communities, I personally strongly believe that more needs to be done. Setting new standards by proactive strategizing and implementation instead of what comes across as reactive. Modern science tells us more than ever that the equilibrium between our brain and body is the most dynamic relationship there is for our brain and physical health. That the direct correlation between the two work together inside the construct of the symbiotic collective of subconscious and conscious states within the mind, that directly affects the body and its function to fight off sickness and disease. This should be reflected in every country's health budgets and efforts to emphasize the counterparts that mental and physical health represent. In Canada the proclaimed budget for Mental Health is around seven percent of the Federal Health Budget. Out of that proclaimed seven percent, I must wonder what percent of that makes it into funding resources and treatment for the public to access? In a country where depression is the leading cause of disease and disability. It would seem to be quite a slap in the face by an ignorant hand of the government and the appointed health officials. Perhaps if they were to open their eyes to truly look at the effects of Mental illness on our nation and dug a little deeper in their overflowing pockets paid by our hard earned tax dollars, it would be fair to say if the percentage of the mental health budget was increased, that the economic "burden" would be decreased as more individuals with Mental illness and Mental Health issues would be more freely able to obtain proper diagnosis and treatment in a reasonable timeframe, as there would be a massive jump in resources and education regarding this "burden." Not for just those affected, but also the potential to increase a positive educational influence among the masses would become a powerful ally in opening the minds of so many of those who do not fully understand the impact of this, and aid in the deconstruction and dissipation of the stigma that blinds so many including many of those in power who have the financial ability to make the necessary changes to our health budgets that are so urgently needed. The CAMH website states "While mental illness accounts for about ten percent of the burden of disease in Ontario, it receives just seven percent of healthcare dollars. Relative to this burden, mental health care in Ontario is underfunded by about $1.5 billion. When compared to its Organization for Economic Co-operation and Development (OECD) counterparts, Canada is well behind other countries that spend ten percent to eleven percent of their health care budgets on mental health." My guess is that an increase to roughly eleven to thirteen percent would balance out the economic burden of mental health and then promote growth on the positive side slowly over time. It would seem to me that the real monster in the shadows is the stigma. I am not an authority on economics, that is just my two cents worth.

I am not a psychologist, psychiatrist, or neurologist. I am not a doctor, nutritionist, or a scientist. I am not a celebrity, a sports icon, or a self-help guru. I am not an expert at anything. I am not going to teach you how to make a million dollars in a month by reading this book. I am not a perfect person. I am not living a perfect life. I am not interested in obtaining sympathy or praise from anyone. I am not always right. I am not without flaws and weaknesses. I am not a typical success story. I am not better than anyone else. This book contains examples of my experiences, perceptions, perspectives, and interpretations of that information.

I am a real person. Just like you. And just like you, I have a story. I believe that sharing our stories is the way to inspire and influence each other. This is my story about how one drop of water had the contingency to end my life or to begin it.

CHAPTER 1

THE END

I know who I am,
The chaos is swarming in my blood.
I can't be anything else.
Blind in darkness,
from the light
I don’t know how to see.
Hospital knives,
can't fix me with surgery
Because you can't save,
The million already dead ghosts inside of me
One last shiver,
Inside a chill
Looking into a mirror,
At the monster I must kill.

NOVEMBER 19TH 2019

I had been sitting on the edge of my couch looking out the window off and on for about an hour. It was a cold, dark and uninviting early November morning. Dark bellied clouds blanketed the sky as far as I could see. It was raining out, not quite cold enough to snow. I was watching the large raindrops fall from the sky in slow motion and then as they hit my window, watching the drops of water slither and snake their way down the glass eventually falling into a small puddle they were forming on my balcony. It was hypnotizing. Teardrops slid slowly down my face in synchronicity.

I was watching an intricately delicate ballet of cohesion and adhesion. A drop of water such as raindrop, teardrop or water drop are all held together by surface tension and all share the course of becoming too heavy and eventually falling from their host due to gravity, whether it be from condensation that gathers on a leaf in the forest and falls to the ground below it. A raindrop falling from an accumulation of vapor and rapid temperature change inside a Cumulonimbus Cloud. A teardrop created from the human eye.

The importance of water drops in our world are preeminent. Binding all life together by being its freshwater life source. Every body of water, big or small, carries an immense purpose in our ecosystems. Puddles, creeks, pools, swamps, marshes, ponds, streams, rivers, lakes, waterfalls, seas, and oceans all are dependent on the mighty raindrop for their existence. Rain being the proprietor, the giver of all life. Without rain and water vapor there would be no life on our planet. The rainfall on the oceans has a profound effect on our weather systems, climate, diluting salts through evaporation and temporarily altering the surface temperatures of the ocean. Obviously, an entire infinite orchestra of water drops are necessary to constantly renew these natural resources, which in turn provide life on land and in all bodies of water.

Every drop of water in a forest or jungle falls from the trees and leaves, landing on the richly organic layer of soils and debris below it. Thus, creating the opportunity for vegetation, fungi, aiding in decomposition of matter and providing plant and tree roots with a nourishing drink. The complex relationship of interaction with all the animals and plants that live there are unique to the biodiversity of its ecosystem, but all rely on water.

A teardrop may not have the significance of providing survival to living things. However, the teardrop has quite an implausible phenomenon unique to human beings. Many other animals have tear ducts just like we do, and their purpose is to provide a liquid to clean irritants from the eye. When dust, dirt, or smoke gets in the eye the tear duct will overflow with lubricant to wash away all irritants, cleansing the eye. A teardrop is composed primarily of water but also contains salt, fatty oils, electrolytes, vitamins, minerals and over fifteen hundred types of proteins.

We are the only animal alive that can generate teardrops through an emotional origin. We shed tears in response to a range of our feelings and emotions. These teardrops contain a higher level of stress hormones than other types. We cry at funerals, when relationships end, when we are saddened or hurt, suffering, but on the same note, we also cry at weddings, when a baby is born, we cry when we laugh uncontrollably, or when we hear or see someone triumph over life threatening odds we rejoice in happy tears. We often feel better after we cry and that is due to shedding emotional teardrops, releases endorphins and oxytocin within the brain. These chemicals make us humans feel good and can ease both emotional and physical pain. Quite the unique spectacle for our species indeed.
Outside my window, I looked at a tree that had been stripped down to nothing from the cold. There was one single brown leaf left on a branch trying desperately to hold on to its life. The cold winds were from the north and gusting, consuming that last bit of hope the leaf had, as it was ripped from the branch and blown away forever.

I closed the blinds on that window and turned around into the darkness of my world. I had shut off all the lights, closed all the blinds on any other windows or doors and disconnected anything that had any form of light shining from it to make it as dark as possible. I had nothing left to see. I did not recognize myself anymore. I had become a ghost. Nobody could see me. I sat down on the floor beside my couch with my back against the wall. The tears I had were very heavy. Heavy with pain. In fact, they were loaded with all the pain I had ever felt in my life inside their composition.

Scattered all over the floor in front of me were letters, poems, and captured thoughts I had written down over the previous days and nights beforehand. I had been drinking for three days and two nights straight. I did not eat. I did not drink any water. Just alcohol, handfuls of sleeping pills and painkillers to slow down and neutralize my over analytical mind. Numbing all the feelings of my memories of my family, friends and loved ones. It was time to finally put an end to the reign of terror from that monster which had controlled my mind since I was a little boy.

I was all alone. Imprisoned inside the walls in my head. Subtle whispers of any hope in the back of my mind that should have sounded as loud as screams for help were quieted by my guilt and shame. The unambiguous symphony of silence was magnified so loud, amplifying the jagged piercing of my own thoughts. The only feeling I had left was pain. My thoughts were marathons of deviation and desperation. My eyes were open, but it was like looking through dark tinted glass. I became monochromatic, even though I remembered how beautiful all the colors of my life once were, I could no longer see them, only felt the void of their absence. My aspirations seemed as pointless as crying into a rapid rushing river and then looking to find my tears downstream. It was like standing outside your own unlocked house in the freezing cold of night, but you don't go inside, because you know that nobody is home. You just stand there, frozen.

The insupportable weight of pressure upon my mind was bleeding out every dream that I have ever had, forcing me to watch in a state of paralysis, as they died an avoidable death. In this world of masquerade, I could see through everyone's mask, seeing who they truly were, yet no one could see me through mine. I was outnumbered by the army of shadows. I was defeated. Unrepairable. I could no longer fight or outrun the monster that lived in the shadows in the corners of my mind. My heart was broken into a million tiny desperate shards like when you throw a bottle against the wall and glass shatters across the floor. The foundation which I was built upon was being washed out by continuous waves composed of self-abandonment, self-betrayal, and self-destruction. I was drowning in the cold waters with no lifeboat in sight. I could feel every person I had let down, hurt physically or emotionally. I had become completely hollowed out and there was nothing left to fill the void inside of me. Desolation. Everything and everyone were gone. I made it all disappear. I had long given up on the idea of someone coming to save me. I had ripped myself open and shown the world who I was, and nobody cared anymore. The pure suffocation of that constricted its grip upon me and I could no longer breathe. The darkest hour had arrived, and it had not come for me in the night. I was trapped inside another world inside of this world. A world without light, without love, without life. The personification of all my abilities, passions, thoughts, ideas, loves, and dreams were all gathered in front of me. They had believed in me wholeheartedly and would have helped me paint the world new colors. Instead, because I never believed in myself, they would all sadly die with me never having the chance to live and flourish. I had sadistically fantasized about this very moment for many years throughout my life. The time had come to execute the monstrosity within and the million different versions of me it had already consumed.

I told myself that the next teardrop that slid down my face and it fell to the floor, that I would end my life. My mind had become a nebulous recollection of my time. It felt like an endless uninhabitable night that would not let the day begin. The darkness disintegrated out the hopes of new daylight. There no longer was a definitive divide between the spaces of life and death. Tears slowly began to form and roll down my face from my bloodshot eyes. They were warm like summer nights on my cold skin. As one paused at the bottom of my jawline, gradually forming the shape of a teardrop, life froze as I understood it, holding time hostage. Perfectly still. A frozen moment where the whole entirety of my life was encapsulated within that one tiny teardrop. All the experiences, memories and events that lead to all my mistakes, failures, heartbreaks, loneliness, fear, anger, self-destruction of my depression was all I felt. I could see all the people I had let down, hurt, or broke their hearts. I could not feel any happy memories whatsoever. No experiences like love, laughter, or joy. They no longer existed in me. It was as though they had been robbed from the bank of my memory. I missed everything that I could not remember. Every single moment of my life began flashing like a strobe light of snapshots. Like a slideshow. Speeding through many of my memories. Some that I had no recollection of, and many that I did. From my birth to my childhood, my teenage years and then my adult life right up to the very moment in which I was trapped in. Reliving literally thousands of experiences at what felt like the speed of light, left my mind spinning and twisting.

I was being serenaded by the echoes of my lost love and the choir of my loneliness. Condemnation cradled my hand as I picked up the gun off the floor beside me. Disengaging the safety sent a shockwave throughout the pin drop silence of my living room. As I put the gun in my mouth the cold bitterness of the metal sent a sensation that felt like ice freezing throughout my veins from my head down to my body. For a brief second, I sat there, calm like a time bomb. Waiting. My mind was finally empty for the first time that I could recall in my entire life. I had finally stopped running away. There I stood, face to face and smirked as I stared into the ravenous eyes of the monster that had been trying to kill me since I was a little boy.

As that teardrop liberated itself and fell from my face suddenly time was released and no longer stood still. Reality hit like a hammer smashing down on the last coffin nail as that one drop of water hit the floor. I took a last deep breath and closed my eyes, kissing the world goodbye. I screamed as loud as I could silently inside my head.

Squeezing the gun handle,
I pulled the trigger.
Blow out the candle.
Darkness

CHAPTER 2

BROOKLYN THE DANCING UNICORN

In my mind I'm a blind man doin' time.
Tupac Shakur

When I was a boy, I often dreamt of inventing a time machine. Partially to escape from the time in which I currently was living in when things got bad, but also to travel throughout time. To go back and see the dinosaurs that I loved to draw and bring to life through my animated imagination. I envisioned them brightly marked, like Poison Dart Frogs. Bold and rich colors with vibrant patterns particular to each species and their prehistoric environments. Far from the drab and lackluster depiction of what Dinosaurs were commonly thought to look like. That bored me. I wanted to visit the future and find a cure for disease and death. So that I could bring it back and share it with the world. As a boy I was very afraid of death. I would make myself sick to my stomach overthinking about what happens after we die. Exploring endless scenarios all night long that had no answers. The concept of eternity was paralyzing and made life seem so pointless. Miniscule on a never beginning or ending timeline.

Almost as if our time was so insignificant that it never even happened. With my imaginary time machine, I wanted to be able to freeze time. To hold it and then expand it. To control it. To have the ability to slow it down in the most amazing moments and to speed through the painful times. I wanted to go back and fix things so that they never happened in the future. Had I known all I needed was a plutonium driven DeLorean for a car and an eccentrically mad scientist for a close friend, my life could have been so different. My time travelling fantasies may have materialized.

Time is such a fascinating concept to me. Our brain is an actual time machine, we can use memory to visit the past and through imagination we can see the future. Time seems to have a variable flex to it. Where one second can feel like a duration as long as a lifetime. Other times the second feels as fast as it truly goes by. It's easy for us to lose track of time when we are distracted, or we are amid challenging our mind. We can become trapped inside a moment in time which dictates the future actions based on the past experiences. Time can stand still, often when we are afraid or scared in a moment of fear it feels like time slows right down, stops and we are frozen. It appears time is not enough when we are excited and, in the chase, pulling out all that we can of that moment. Inside the brain where time is truly constructed and uncontrolled. There is no true timeline. The brain is doing so many functions being charged by electrical movements, neurons firing in many directions like fireworks, managing millions of sensory and involuntary actions, time doesn't matter to the brain. it's not an important element to its function. However, the mind obviously works within the constructs of time that we have created for ourselves. Like if we are trying to complete a task or make a deadline, or understand why something's taking so long, or the simplicity of our memory.

Dyschronometria is the condition of distorted time perception. Making it difficult to assess how much time has taken place. I believe that we all have similarities to this condition throughout our lives. Perhaps not as drastic as those who experience this condition due to the cerebellar dysfunction. Be that as it may, some things feel as though they just took place even though the experience happened many years ago. Time has this fascinating elasticity to it. Flexibility that can be stretched by our minds. In a life-threatening situation our minds slow down time which alters our cognitive reality. It appears the tempo of external life has the effect of compression or expansion of how long something lasts. Meaning that the tempo of our eternal experiences has an impact on the internal reality of the timeline in our conscious minds. As we age, it seems as though time quickens. That time happens faster. When we were kids, time was simpler, less memories to cloud the brain. Playing outside for an hour when completely cognitively immersed in imagination would seem endless and uninterrupted. Time felt like it stood still.

Our inner chronometry is dictated by the elastic properties of memory shaping. Time controls memory and memory shapes the experience of our time. This is the genesis of time perception. Time is perceived in two ways, prospectively and retrospectively. Now and then. This is how we can estimate time and gauge it accordingly.

It would seem to me that there is a tightrope walk between the equilibrium of the brain and the mind regarding the relevance of time. Losing balance on that tight rope and shifting too far one way could dramatically change the perception of time. I wondered what it would be like if the brain voluntarily took over time in the consciousness of my mind. Would time stand still? Would it feel differently? Would the value of the duration of time still hold meaning in relevance to experiences without the emotional attachment of my distinct memory? Is it possible that the physical realm of time could be lost inside the dimension of conscious time?

This is when someone should have warned me to be careful what you wish for.

Was I dead? I was trapped inside the abyss of my mind. Every direction I looked there was darkness as far as I could see. All around me. All above me. I could feel the pressure of its vastness all upon me. It was terrifying, yet I felt inanimate inside that moment in time, lost somewhere in the labyrinth of my mind. It was cold, empty, an endless void. It felt like I was trapped inside a massive ocean of emptiness but also it felt so tiny and contained. The pressure of all the darkness around me began to increase and it became suffocating.

Calmly crushing me. No matter how hard I tried to fight against it, it just kept coming for me. I screamed for help but there was nobody that could hear me. I just heard the ongoing echo of my scream bounce around until it eventually faded away. In the far distance behind me, I could hear the bellowing roar of the monster ripping through the void as it was getting closer every time I called out for help. The darkness was wrapping itself around me, strangling me. Seconds felt like days trapped inside an eternally dark abyss. Time was warped. Enclosed inside what seemed to be an infinite moment that offered no sign of ending or beginning. Like being in another dimension where the boundaries of time did not exist.

Far off in the distance ahead of me, there was a tiny moving silhouette in the eclipse of the shadow from what seemed to be a sliver of flickering light coming towards me. Its presence made me begin to feel anxious, scared, but at the same time suspiciously spellbound. As it moved closer to me, I started trying to look and understand what this little blurry shimmer of light that was dancing in front of me. Unexpectedly, I could hear what sounded like a young child laughing and giggling. I could feel the vibrations of the sounds. The closer it got to me I began to focus and see a young little girl with strawberry blonde hair, big crystal blue eyes, she was wearing a brightly colored unicorn headband complimented with a slate blue princess dress with clear but sparkly butterfly wings on the back of it. She began skipping and dancing around me. She was laughing and her laugh sounded so familiar. She was in and out of focus with a circumambient glow. I was so confused by all of this. Was I alive, was I dead, was my mind playing some sort of trick on me? Was this a transition from life to death? Was this limbo or purgatory? Why wasn't she scared like I was? In the wake of that exact moment, the young girl walked right up to me. Looked at me dead in the eyes, in sort of a humorous cute mocking gesture with her hands on her hips. She asked me this in a matter-of-fact way... "Why are you here?" I was absolutely taken back by her question as it echoed, I began tearing up as she waited for my response. I could not speak. I was frozen in complete shock. Words were just too heavy and hard to say. The little girl fidgeted and swayed her head from side to side as if her body language was telling me to hurry up and answer. "What are you doing?" She asked. Her question was so innocent, but so challenging as it exposed the reality of the situation. I said to the little unicorn girl in a choked-up voice "I'm so sorry sweetheart, but I can't tell you that. Not right now. I'm so sorry." She bounced back and forth for a second or two, and then looked at me again with a wide-eyed puzzled look upon her face and asked, "where are you going?" Everything went numb with the realization of the acknowledgement of what I had done. It was like that pitiful feeling of disappointing someone you loved badly; I did not know what to say. My words got too hard to speak. I could not talk. As I was about to attempt to reply to her, I started crying instead of talking. My hands were trembling and too heavy to lift. I could not hide my face or tears from her. That is when the little dancing unicorn took my hand in hers and looked up at me and smiled with her big blue eyes and said "Jay McLean, you can't go, you can't go." And then, in the blink of an eye, she was gone, expeditiously vanishing back into that tiny sliver of flickering light.

It was in that very moment, that millisecond inside the time warp of my mind, that I could see everything. It was like watching an electrical storm in the sky. Bright colorful flashes of lightning dancing across from cloud to cloud. And then it flashed so bright, like a thunderbolt hit me. All I could see was endless light from an explosion that rocked the whole entirety of me. It was like looking at all the stars in the universe at the darkest time of night. A billion molecular dissections of everything that I was composed of. Every singular thought, idea, feeling and memory. In the very boundless wonder of all of what I was seeing, a number of very specific and precise images were burned so brightly into my memory. Like I was a blindman seeing for the first time. Catching a frog, a guinea pig, peanut butter packets on a table in a restaurant, a dark mountain range, a barracuda swimming in the ocean, a pile of sticks and stones, a pair of pants on fire, a spoonful of honey, a monarch butterfly, a chameleon changing its colors, scars on my body, sitting on the floor of an empty gym, a samurai warrior, my reflection in rear view mirror and a waterfall.

Then suddenly, as quickly as everything that just took place, without warning all the light began being vacuumed backwards to its origin like it was caught inside a black hole in outer space. Being sucked back so instantaneously. Like watching a movie on rewind at the highest speed imaginable. Then as fast as it all happened, it was over, it all went black. Returning me to darkness.

In the distance, I could hear a faint and muffled ring going off every half second. It became intensely louder with each succession. Like an alarm clock going off inside my head. I realized that it was a phone ringing. I started trying to focus on the sound coming from the phone and then BOOM. Like a gunshot so loud that it jolted my body, like I was waking up from in an eclectic chair.

That's when my eyes opened. In utter disarray, confusion, and shock, I looked out at my surroundings. Taking a huge gulp of air. Like I had been drowning underwater and then somehow finally surfaced and took that lifesaving breath. Even though it was dark in the room, it was so bright that it hurt my eyes. That snapped me out of my dreamlike state. I looked down at my right hand, which was holding the gun. Like a flash flood, feelings began crashing through me. I would imagine that there was a look of absolute terror on my face. In my mind a surge of thought and emotion. I exhaled my breath over and over, each time louder than the previous. I did not comprehend what was going on. All these things that I could not explain to myself at that time were swirling around inside my head like a tornado. Rational thought was an obscure concept. I slowly turned around to the wall behind me, expecting to see my blood and brain matter plastered all over the wall. Like some atrocious abstract piece of sadistic art but the wall was blank. Clean. Normal. Unaffected. I was in such disbelief. Was this some sort out of body experience like many others have claimed to have had when dying. Was this my mind playing more tricks on me? It all felt like being submerged in a dream-like state of suspended animation, where I was just beginning to wake up, but I was still asleep. My phone rang again. This time it startled me. Kickstarting my brain back into action. That's when the bareknuckle truth of reality punched me. Waking me up to the realization that I was still alive. That I had failed in taking my life. I was in a state of shock. How? Was this some practical joke from the universe? Failure was the cause of my demise and now failure has become the genesis of life. It seems I had been slapped in the face by the hand of irony.

I folded in half, like a jack knife on my floor. The guilt of my failed suicide was too much for me. I began to feel every single person's pain and suffering that would have been affected by my death. I could feel their tears. Their heartache. The catastrophic trauma it would have caused my family and close friends. I felt my sisters trying to hold it together while they attempted numerous times to explain to their kids why I was gone. How it would have torn my parents apart. Destroying them. Leaving them with nothing but an onslaught of pain and never-ending questions that there would never be answers to. Devastating my friends with the everlasting guilt that they didn't do enough for me or weren't there when I needed them. Many people left with only the questions of why didn't he ask for help? Why didn't he talk to me and tell me what was going on with him?

I was spinning out of control. I felt so bad but at the same time I felt unsettled, unfinished. I was furious that I failed my mission to end my pain and stop running from the monster in the shadows. But every time I began to obsess about taking my life again, my thoughts shifted unconsciously to that little dancing unicorn girl's questions. Why am I here? What am I doing? Where am I going?

To which I had no answers.

My phone was ringing again, and I was getting notifications of text messages. I was reluctant to look at my phone. Mortified, in fact. I did not want to face the potent palpability of actuality that embodied the situation in front of me. I walked to my bathroom and looked in the mirror. I did not recognize the person I was looking at. What I saw in my reflection was a scared little boy trapped inside my body. I saw conflict. A war that had been raging on my entire life between who I really was, and who I was trying to pretend to be. There were casualties on both sides. No one was winning, both sides were losing. I saw a little boy that would cry out for attention and then turn away and run as soon as he got it. I saw a man that got all the attention, but it was never enough to make up for what he lost as a boy. I remember looking at my reflection and asking, "why are you here?" Again, I had no answer.

As I sat down on my couch, I exhaled powerfully. My mind was still very foggy and my thoughts insatiably erratic. I was still having a tremendous difficulty in understanding the gravity of my current situation. My focus turned to the little dancing unicorn that had somehow entered my mind in the most astonishing way. How was that even possible? Was it my brain or mind's last attempt to save me? To distract me. To bring me back. Had my brain shut down in preparation to preserve itself before anticipating the gun blast and was this the state of consciousness of my mind that had remained afterwards? Why was it her and not someone else? The most remarkable element of all of this was that I knew her. I knew the little dancing unicorn well. Her name is Brooklyn, she was five years old at the time, the daughter of my closest and dearest friends.

The same friends who had been calling and texting me repeatedly. That little dancing unicorn saved my life that day. If it wasn't for her and her questions, somehow subconsciously entering my mind state at that exact moment, I may not still be here. She will always be my hero for the rest of my living years.

Three of my good friends from work texted me as I obviously did not show up that morning. They sent some chirps poking fun at me. Making references to how hard I must have partied that weekend. It brought a smirk to my face despite the dilemma, as these chirps were perfectly aligned with the characteristic comedy in our daily conversations.

Another good friend whose daughter Kiera is my biggest fan, had called and messaged me as well out of concern. Kiera who was three years old at that time would have her mama record her telling me "She loved me and missed me" and then had her mom send it to me. Sometimes the tiniest little voice can be the one of loudest songs on the soundtrack of saving someone's life.

I responded by text message to all those who had messaged or called me. Replying with the same message to all, that I was not feeling well and tired, just not feeling myself and that I was sorry if I had caused any worry. I did not want to burden anyone with the weight of the truth of my predicament. I still felt very lost inside the maze of indifference of my volatile mind. I did manage to write down all the distinct images that were brightly burnt into my memory as my brain had kick started back to life. Catching a frog, a guinea pig, peanut butter packets on a table in a restaurant, a dark mountain range, a barracuda swimming in the ocean, a pile of sticks and stones, a pair of pants on fire, a spoonful of honey, a monarch butterfly, a chameleon changing its colors, scars on my body, sitting on the floor of an empty gym, a samurai warrior, my reflection in a rear-view mirror and a waterfall. I needed to know why these images were so prominently illustrated in that experience. What did they mean? Why were they significant? I lied on the cold floor, staring off into what seemed like an out of focus blurred kaleidoscope as the room started to spin, and like a broken record, I kept repeating to myself "I'm sorry" over and over for what seemed like an eternity, until my eyes gently closed at last, the hamster wheel stopped spinning and the lights finally went out.

CHAPTER 3

HOME ALONE

A season of isolation and loneliness is when the caterpillar gets its wings. Remember that next time you feel alone.
Mandy Hale

In the days, weeks and months that followed my suicide attempt I was still battling my depression every day. I hated being alone. Alone with my thoughts. I could not handle the reality of the world I was living in. It was like two worlds were colliding. One was a world that should have ended and the other was a world that was just beginning. The contemplation of taking my life was still lingering around in the dark shadows of my mind. I was fixating on all the negative narratives of my current situation. Not changing anything regarding the way I approached my day. At best, I was going through the motions like an automated robot. I would go to work even though I hated it there, just so I did not have to be alone. I did like being around my co-workers. After work I would go to a neighborhood restaurant and sit at the bar usually by myself and have a few pints talking with the staff that had become like a small family to me. They were kind enough to listen to me ramble on about whatever was on my mind. They cared about me and that meant so much more than any of them probably knew at that time. They laughed at my bad jokes which I had an arsenal of. There were other regulars that I would see often there and every once and awhile I would chat with them too depending what mood I was in. From that bar top, I established a couple good new friendships. I would usually be dressed in a suit, looking very sharp. Part of my disguise, part of the masquerade. A deceptional masterpiece.

I wanted a better life for myself, but I was unable to see past the wall of self-designed apocalyptic prophecies that held me back from moving forward. Inauspiciously condemned to be chained to my fears of being alone. At that time, I did not want to understand why I feared being alone, instead I would just continue to avoid being alone with my thoughts as much as possible and by any means necessary. Always on the run. Inevitably, that shotgun blast was never too far behind me.

There is a saying that goes "if you can't make it, fake it." I acted accordingly and fulfilled that advice throughout the holidays in the following month of December. I was so drained and lifeless inside but put on my happy face for my family and friends as best I could, even though I hated it. Everything felt counterfeit. I wanted nothing to do with anyone over the holidays. Things were getting really bad inside my head again. The shadows were beginning to march, and the commencement of creeping thoughts were gaining strength. The stress of being broke over the holidays was difficult to endure when it came time for gifts. The pain of feeling broken was hard to conceal. I had given up all hope and attempted to take my life only a month earlier and my family had no idea, while I sat there fighting back tears. Pretending to be okay. I wanted to ask them for help, but I did not want to interrupt Christmas. I felt like a burden. Why couldn't I just grow up and be normal like everybody else. I was supposed to be a grown man, yet I was still a child. Boys don't cry.

A month or so later, in January and then into February of 2020, the whole world blew up. A shockwave of fear felt around the planet created in the media about another new deadly virus that would annihilate us all had become the center of attention. The horrific and terrifying tales of the projections that this unknown virus was going to rip through the population and have massively catastrophic consequences. The sun lit sky was torched with fear and left behind an ominous cloud of uncertainty structured with forecasts of gloom and doom. It was like everybody stopped looking for the sun and instead instantly directed all their attention to darkened opaque overcast. Obscuring the clarity of many of the population's perception as more confusing and conflicting information regarding this virus was created by the media and governments around the world. It appears every news station, newspaper, media outlet and social media platforms were bombarding the public with an onslaught of dictated narratives focusing only on all the negatives of the virus. Pounding into the minds of people to be very scared, to isolate and to wear masks to be safe from the rampant spread of this new mystery virus. A pandemic status was created responsible for sending the world into a spiral of overactive dumbfounded behavior. Toilet paper was bought in bulk and hoarded to ensure survival of the fittest of our species. A shining moment of glory in the process of natural selection, truly representing the intellectual dominance of our genotype.

At the end of February, I got sick. Throughout my life I have succumbed to recurrent pneumonia several times causing some issues with my lungs. I developed chronic bronchitis throughout the latter portion of my childhood and continued to be affected by that throughout my life. Usually, every year I would typically get sick for a couple weeks after my birthday which is at the end of February. Perhaps the many long hours of darkness and shortened daylight had a seasonal effect on my immune system. Concurrently, I would also feel very depressed around this time of the year. Cold winter temperatures presented a harsh climate to be socially active in. Due to the ongoing frenzy about this mystery virus, I was forced to quarantine and isolate for fourteen days. I lived alone and the idea of not being able to go anywhere or see anyone was very inconvenient and uncomfortable to say the least. I had a deep barking cough, felt weak and tired but did not have a fever or any of the main symptoms of the new virus. Regardless, I was still sick and if I coughed out in public people would look at me like I was a murderer. My fear of being alone was about to unwillingly become the forefront of my attention and not being able to constantly distract myself by always being out and about places was coming to a very abrupt end.

As the next weeks went on, the government decided to close gyms, restaurants, bars, label, and separate people as essential or non-essential workers, cancel all large social gatherings except for the ones inside big box stores. These American owned overpopulated stores were a safe haven from the virus, but small local businesses were not according to the logical leadership of the government. Small businesses were targeted as a direct threat to spreading the infection rate and had to close their doors immediately. Panic was encouraged by the media's relentless focus on the deaths and infection rate of this flu-like virus. I often pondered why they did not focus on the astronomically high survival rate of people who were not already dying of multiple illnesses or were under the age of eighty-five that had come in contact with it.

The rest of the city began to shut down in a government mandated lockdown. Therefore, extending the period of my isolation. I had been completely alone for over two weeks at that point already. Not being able to see my family or friends, co-workers, go to the gym or anywhere else for that matter. I was still dealing with a lingering hacking cough but was on the mend.

I had started taking some anti-depressant medication prescribed from my doctor just after New Year's Day. The medication would help stabilize my moods by modifying the chemicals in my brain and increase neurotransmitters like Norepinephrine and Dopamine. Effective treatment for major depression disorder. It was a time-released drug that I found helpful in the early stages of my recovery. It seemed to be beneficial in keeping me level during the acclimatization stages of my initial inauguration of isolation. That would be put to the test as one night I was awoken to my phone ringing and alerting me of text messages around 3:45 am. It was both my sisters calling and texting me to inform me that my dad had been rushed to the emergency at a hospital in an ambulance. As I started to get ready to go to the hospital, I messaged my sister who was there with him, to tell her I was on my way. She explained to me that I was not allowed in the hospital due to the restrictions put in place and that I could not go there because I was sick. At that point in time my father was unable to be stabilized by the medical staff as there were issues with his blood sugar levels being so low. They were checking to see if his brain was bleeding or if he had a stroke due to his mannerisms and actions. I became very upset and in fact furious. I remember asking my sister the gut-wrenching question of if he was going to die would I not be allowed to be there to hold his hand and tell him that I love him as he passed on, the answer was no, I would not be allowed to do that. Sadly, my father had been in and out of the hospital quite frequently with many complications over the past decade and it was always painful to see him in there. The amount of anger and frustration that was brooding because I could not be by his side when he needed me most became irrepressible. I relied on text messages for any updates on my dad's condition. The time between messages felt like a test of my mental endurance. I was not passing this test. My thoughts began wandering into the twisted realm of worst-case scenarios. Overthinking has always been one of my worst enemies. To the point where I have lost control of the thoughts being produced in my mind.

As the day went on and the time seemed to drag on so slowly that it stood still, finally after approximately twelve hours, I received the news that my father had been stabilized. They had ruled out a brain bleed or stroke after the results of the CT scan came back negative. He would spend another four days in the hospital and then return home. I was relieved that he was doing better but at the same time I was struggling with the reality of the restrictions imposed due to this virus. It was like getting stuck in quicksand. The more I struggled with it, the more it slowly pulled me down. Side note: Quicksand should be called slow sand and it is impossible to die in it, as the density of the sand is greater than that of our body. It's basically sand that act like a liquid due to saturation and is rarely deeper than a few feet. You can get stuck in it and gradually sink a bit if one was to move frequently. Causing an inconvenience at best. A far cry from the TV shows and Movies I grew up watching where it seemed as though quicksand was literally everywhere, threatening the life of humans who somehow unwillingly got trapped in the deadly pits of it. I suppose one less thing in life to worry about.

I drank heavily that night, my way of coping with the turmoil of the state of my compromised mental health. When I woke up the next morning, I was hungover and very depressed. I was still sick with my bronchial infection and felt like garbage. Throughout the day I would begin to obsess on all the negative things that I could cram into my head all at once. Creating a tsunami wave of destructive force that obliterated any rational thoughts. I quickly began reliving past events that I felt out of control of. Forcing redundant emotions to surface. My anxiety of the uncertain future combined with my depression of my past created a whirlpool that I was drowning in. Cold violent waters in which my thoughts encircled inside my mind. Twisting and turning. As the day turned into the evening, my mental state worsened. Menacing and frantic assessments and conclusions of the way I was feeling only added to the momentum of the negative energies surrounding me. My thoughts were racing wildly out of my control. I began having difficulty breathing, I was at times unable to catch my breath. My heart was pounding like I had just narrowly escaped a near death experience. It felt like someone had ripped open a hornet's nest in my guts. I was in a panicked state of fear. Hyperventilating on my floor. I could not slow down my thoughts or control my emotions. The constant fear of being alone and isolated for the rest of my life became claustrophobic as it seemed everything was closing in on me and time was running out. My mental breakdown got worse, and I was flooded with suicidal thoughts, like the ones I had only a few months before. I was in dire need of help but refused to call 911. I was friends with a few firefighters, and they were the first responders to emergency calls, and I did not want anyone I knew to see me like that. I did not want to be taken to a hospital either. My ego was holding the reins and in control. I was too arrogant and pretentious in the moment when I needed to ask for help.

I called one of my sisters out of desperation and in the very moment when she answered the phone and heard my voice, she knew something was dreadfully wrong. As we spoke for a minute or two, her first immediate recommendation was to call an ambulance which I absolutely refused even though it felt like I was on the verge of going into cardiac arrest. In hindsight, it's truly incredible what the mind can trigger your body to do in response to the state of fear in your mind. Over the course of the next hour and a half my sister would gradually talk me down. Calming my mind by continuously reminding me that these thoughts were just thoughts and not what was really happening. That it was temporary and would not last forever. She helped slow the spin cycle by concentrating on helping me control my breathing. She told me that it was ok to feel the way I did, but she also helped me to realize that I was going to make it out of that mental breakdown alive. We worked on a plan together that would help me get through the rest of the night if the recurrence of my negative forecasting was to present itself again. I told myself over and over that I would not live-in fear anymore for the rest of the night until I fell asleep.

The following morning is when everything in my life changed. I woke up a man on a mission. An awakening. No more feeling sorry for myself. No more excuses. No more blame. No more victimizing. No more sitting around waiting for something to happen. No more fear. I made the decision to go all in and re-calibrate all my energy into resisting the seduction of past emotions that had held me captive within the prison cell in the dark shadows of my mind.

It had become obvious to me that I was in a fight or flight response to situations I was in, and I have always previously been a fighter. I had given up temporarily in the defeat I believed to be true inside my head. That weakened state would prove to be the catalyst of the greatest strength I have ever known in myself. It would become the reference point of all my changes. Supplying a boundless amount of motivation in which I would draw from and continue faithfully throughout my odyssey. I had my starting point established and was ready to get back in the ring and start fighting again.

As I enjoyed my morning coffee, I began writing. I wrote myself a letter. In that letter I apologized to myself for giving up on life previously and declared to myself that would not be allowed to take place ever again. I wrote that I promised myself an undying commitment to change. That I would confront all my fears no matter how hard that might be. I would dedicate whatever it took to breaking through all the chains from my past that were holding me back in the present moments. I wrote that I would spend as much time as I could learning about who I was and how I could improve the areas that needed positive adjustments. That I would study the mind, the brain, psychology, anything related to how my thoughts and emotions worked so I could gain a better understanding to plan for my growth. I needed to become as knowledgeable as I possibly could in relation to mental illness and mental health through intransigent analysis. In concluding the letter to myself, I stated that I was excited to get to know myself better and help myself become everything that I have always wanted to be. Freeing myself from my own trap of punishment. I still read the letter often as it is a wonderful roadmap from where I once was to where I am now.

We often get caught up in the long view of what change looks like. We visualize all the things we believe have to take place to make a change becoming an arduous endeavor. The focal point is wrongly placed on the long-drawn-out scenario we create in our minds about making the change. I can personally assure anyone that change happens as fast as a snap of the fingers from my own experience. Change happens the second we just go for it. Literally everything changed as soon as I believed it would and took the necessary actions to support that blindfolded way of thinking. A leap of faith in self. Was my life instantly perfect? No, not even remotely close and it remains as a work in progress today. But it did get better. Every minute I was dedicating myself to self-improvement would set me up for the next opportunity to grow into the next necessary action. I started writing down everything. I wanted to put all of everything I was onto paper so I could read it over and examine all the details. Some of the largest explanations were tiny possessions of treasured information hidden within the smallest of details. Immediately exposing connections from one detail to the next. In the beginning it was disorganized chaos as I wrote down whatever came to mind but it felt real and organic in its flow and so I left it uninterrupted and raw. Systematically over the next few weeks of isolation I would begin to categorize my writing into an inventory-like arrangement. As well I began getting up early in the morning. I would wake up before the sun came up and drink a glass of water. Stretch for a few minutes and then regardless of the weather, I was out the door for a run. For the record I would like to state that I utterly detested running. Especially on an empty stomach first thing in the often-cold darkness of the early morning. But that is why I did it every single day.

Freezing temperatures, snow, rain, howling winds or whatever it was did not stop me. It became a challenge to push myself past my limits of mental and physical comfort. Stretching the barriers of my mind. I turned everything into an internal competition. Every morning I had to run fast and far enough to make it to a certain point on the path that I ran on every day, so that the sun would rise behind me, letting me know that the universe had my back and that I was indeed on the right path at the right time in my life. The competition was that every morning the sun came up a bit earlier, meaning I had to get up earlier every new day to ensure success. When I would return home from my daily competition, I was full of ambition and enthusiasm for the day ahead of me. Locomotion caused quite the commotion within the state of my emotion. Movement generates momentum. After I crushed my run, I would perform mental exercises for a couple hours like my take on meditating, or reading, as well as listening to all types of people who I found to be very inspiring, sharing the particulars about their stories. Then the writing would begin. I would target specific areas of my life that I knew needed some tender loving care, dedication to attention and self-administered tough love. The prompt changes that took place in my perspective were defined by the actions in which I chose how to see things. Meaning that when I chose to look at the specifics of what I had written down on paper open mindedly, accompanied with the vision that I was being presented with an opportunity of higher understanding of self whether what was written was good or bad, I was thankful for it. This newly acquired action would change the outcome of everything into a positive regardless of whatever it was because it modified the navigation of my thoughts.

As I spent more time totally alone in isolation, amazing miracles took place every day in my new life. Without my newly adopted change in perspective, I would have been blind and not have been able to see these miracles as the negative outlook I had been so accustomed to would have easily overlooked them. I believed that every new day was a new life. Within the new life I was able to not only confront the fears that had previously controlled me, but I was also able to learn from them. I remember chatting with people and explaining to them about my daily routines and I was often asked about why in the world would I get up as early as I did to be alone as long as possible every single day. The answer was because I was facing my greatest fears. The fear of being alone, the fear of failure and the fear of the unknown. The only way that I envisioned beating my depression and freeing myself from the grips of the dark spirit of the shadow monster was to defeat it was by vanquishing what held me back from doing so all those years. The more time spent alone with my thoughts and emotions, the more time I had to make sense of the experiences that had shaped me as a person and then to celebrate existing good habits while exploring ideas of how to change negative habits from my past into great habits of the present and future. I looked for the origins of my pre-established behaviors from the experiences of my past so that I would be able to be conscious of them while assembling a battle plan. A battle-ready plan for growth and advancement. I would unlearn and relearn so many things in this process.

After being completely alone for over an entire month with the only occasional social interaction I had being with the cashiers at the grocery store, I was getting stronger in so many ways. Every day I was in absolute silence from the moment I woke up until I went to bed unless I was listening to an educational or inspirational resource such as a podcast, audiobook, or a speech. I had implemented a daily structure of consistent routine that I found to work extremely well. Wake up before sunrise. Get out of bed instantly and smile as big as I could no matter how I felt. This set the introductory positive mood for the day. Drink water, but not just any old water. I drank warm water with lemon and Himalayan Sea salt, and I drank it down as quickly as possible. Himalayan salt is harvested from a dried-up sea in Pakistan and is not polluted with manmade chemicals and is very high in potassium which balances the sodium. Once dissolved in warm water the salt creates ions which are exceptional for neurological, cardiovascular, muscular, and cellular health. The lemon adds flavor and helps alkaline levels in the body creating an energy rush. Run outside and beat the sunrise while listening to uplifting and motivational content. Overcoming a hard task first thing in the day that would raise my feel-good chemicals in my brain and the activity would empower me for the day ahead. Return home and put on coffee and then shower, finishing with freezing cold water for a minimum of thirty seconds. Another test of will which was difficult and uncomfortable but always left me feeling invigorated and very awakened. Meditation for ten minutes, calming my mind and clearing out the overly cluttered nonsensical thoughts that I no longer needed attachment to. Learning to focus my mind and breathing was a challenge everyday as my ADHD loved to run a quarterback blitz on this play. New challenges meant new ways to blueprint alternative methods. Coffee with honey and some ice cubes to cool it down and write out my battle plan for the day. A list of tasks, activities, challenges, and amendments that would provide a strengthening and bonding practice of understanding and the implementation of newfound knowledge about myself. Read for twenty minutes or so, reflecting on what I had learned from whatever book or article I was reading. Write about subjects in accordance with the proclaimed daily battle plan for about two hours. Workout for one hour to two hours. Incorporating body weight exercises such as wide grip pull ups, chin ups, pushups, squats, handstand pushups, and dips. I added kickboxing and yoga into the mix. Resistance training with bands. All done to the point of mental and physical exhaustion. I ate my first meal of the day after being awake and active for five hours which was usually around nine in the morning which consisted of fruits and vegetables accompanied by a source of protein. I researched which fruits and vegetables benefited the stabilization of mood and reduced the symptoms of depression. My favorites included apples, blueberries, kiwis, grapefruit, bananas, oranges, cucumber, and spinach which I prefer to pronounce as spinooch because I like to live on the edge. I often snuck in chocolate chip cookies that I would bake the evening before as a favorite morning snack. Pro tip, dip them in natural peanut butter.

On one day into my transformation, I decided to conduct an autopsy on myself. An autopsy is an examination performed to determine the cause of death or to gain understanding of a disease and how it affected the body. I wanted to do the same for myself even though I was still alive. I wanted to go back to the moment when I attempted to take my life and examine my state of mind and mental health, my thoughts and emotions that were involved and how the disease of mental illness was mechanically involved. So, I cut myself wide open. Exposing everything that I was made of. Figuratively speaking of course. Documenting what I could on pieces of blank white paper that I would eventually post up on my walls of a spare room so that I could visually take in and comprehend all the connections from each piece of paper that represented a little slice of me being that of an experience, an emotion, or a behavior. This would unveil actions and reactions that were thought processes that had become my habits. This matrix-like network of my inner connections of all that made up my personality would span around all four walls in my spare bedroom once completed. An elaborately decorated atlas of the illustrated world inside the immense constellations of my mind surrounded me as I sat in the middle of it all and marveled at the limitless possibilities that were all lighting up all around me. Every piece of paper was connected to every other piece of paper by an origin of an experience, or an emotional state caused by an experience, but also presented many encouraging possibilities to gain insight into how to flip all the negatives into positives just by choosing how I perceived the experience and the contingency it offered me to learn from. I had inadvertently created a Youniverse specific to my life through being an imagineer. The combination of engineering new thoughts and applying action to them while conceiving new alternative outcomes through my imagination made this all come to life just like the big bang theory. An explosive combustion of a creative entity. Granting me the ability to warp and shape my own reality in a future tense through the power of belief. I believed it and therefore I could see it, whereas before, I had to see it, to believe it as most people do. Meaning that what I envisioned for myself in the future became like a memory before it even happened by simply attaching emotion to it and feeling that projection as though it had already happened. You are what you think. Your thoughts become your reality. Your energy through action attracts what you envision. Manifestation is an authentically miraculous superpower

Isolation had become my best friend. My companion. It provided me with the circumstances that helped me to take responsibility for my life. To accept where I was and learn how to navigate through my depression to where I wanted to be. Inquisitively sparking my mind to question everything about myself and my life in a non-cynical way but instead in a perpetual state of wonder. I was able to understand what caused all the fears in my life and how they had shaped my behaviors over the years through the autopsy I performed. Isolation exposed the truths that I had been too scared to face for far too long and from that experience I was able to formulate strategies that would become effective daily, weekly, monthly, and yearly battle plans that would ignite the torches of innovation and change. The combination of all these miracles that materialized during isolation would offer me something that I had never ever truly had before. Purpose. A radical addition to the many newfound alterations to the design of who I was becoming. Through the devotion of routine self-discipline, I spearheaded newfangled self-respect that in turn opened the entrance to the revolving door to self-love. This transformation would become a model that I would implement regarding all aspects of my life. A triad of transformation that was responsible for the inception of my purpose. My purpose radiated clarity. Pioneering the groundbreaking and world-shaking revolution within. I needed to give back to this life, to this world. I wanted to change the world and I believed that was my purpose. Sanctifying this belief and declaring all my efforts to it at whatever cost.

Simultaneously due to the mandated lockdown or quarantine, I wanted to come up with something immediately to help people feel better and laugh even though the cloud of uncertainty hung low in the sky. The overall mood was dark, and people were depressed. Jobs and businesses were in question of remaining intact, social interaction was frowned upon and not allowed; people were beginning to feel desperate. I had to come up with something that I could use to reach people and help change their demeanor. I would use my social media to be the platform to do this. Enter Steve.

Steve is my aloe vera plant that I comically referred to as my roommate. I wrote up several sketches that I would film in hopes that I could make my friends laugh at. I basically made a fool of myself by telling my plant Steve bad dad jokes in the attempt to make my plant do the impossible which was breaking his silence and laughing out loud at my awful jokes while at the same time I would dramatically overreact to my plants silence and refusal to cooperate. I posted the first video, and I expected a few friends and some acquaintances to make fun of me but at the same time hopefully to get a laugh out of it. This was a subtle beta test as I wanted to see if I could positively influence other people through being vulnerable and putting myself out there. I wanted to change how people were feeling. The results would blow my mind. Mind bottling. Over the course of the next two days, I would receive close to two thousand messages from people on my social media and to my phone. A few concerned people had asked if I had lost my mind in which I happily responded yes to. Most of the messages were people thanking me for the video. That it had provided a comical distraction from the gloomy circumstances that they were in. That the laughs were greatly appreciated and just what they needed. I also had a significant number of very heartfelt messages as well from people who were struggling in isolation. Sharing with me the story of their grim situations and how the video helped them by interrupting the twisting thoughts they were having. This brought tears to my eyes as I responded to them because it was the realization that my ideas and intentions were surpassing what I had envisioned and was securing the embodiment of my purpose. My purpose, to help influence other people for the greater good, using my story and articulating the vulnerability of my experiences in the hopes of changing the world, one mind at a time. Purpose is only possible with belief. I believe this more with every new breath I take. For those who are not yet fighters I want to remind you that you are still here and that means you are still in the fight. Your time will come, and you will find your strength through your weaknesses just like I did. Everything you have done up to this point makes you a fighter and don't forget that.

For the first time in my life, I was happy to be alone. I no longer felt loneliness or was afraid of being alone with my thoughts. In isolation I was able to put myself on a path of self-discovery in which I would be a trailblazer. Connecting all the trails through the unexplored wilderness of my lifetime that would lead me to the uncharted area of my purpose. Isolation chartered the autopsy of self which revealed the connections from all the very distinct images that were burnt into my mind when regaining consciousness after my suicide attempt and the equivalence to the corresponding experiences that manifested into the chapters of my life story. By pushing myself past my mental, emotional, and physical barriers in my daily regimen of discipline, I stumbled upon the most beautiful thing I had ever seen. The opportunity to become who I was meant to be.

I am happy to report that Steve is alive and well and still has not laughed at any of my jokes. Not yet.

There was another miracle that came from the guide to the galaxies of my mind, experiences and life mapped all around that spare bedroom. As I swiveled on a bar stool that I sat on in the middle of it all, that lightning bolt hit me in the brain again. Brilliantly exposing the intertwined relevance of all the mysterious images that were so vividly unveiled to me that I had previously written down months before, just after my brain fired back up from my suicide attempt. I saw and understood how each of those images connected to experiences in my life. Those experiences shaped the distinctive uniqueness of my life. Each part of my life had a story within the bigger story. How could a chameleon changing its color, catching a frog or a barracuda swimming in the ocean be related to the makeup of my personality traits? Or a pair of pants on fire? A spoonful of honey? The answers became obvious to me. It was like looking up at the uninterrupted sea of endless stars on a clear dark night and finding the patterns among the constellations that are recognizable such as the Big Dipper, Orion's belt, or Ursa Major (the great bear). Tying it all in together and making sense of the Youniverse to which I found myself centered in. Displaying to me the way home and the remarkable expedition of my trials and tribulations that awaited me.

CHAPTER 4

CATCHING FROGS

It's not easy being green.
Kermit the Frog

When I was a young boy my absolute favorite thing to do was to go catch frogs. In early spring as soon as the sun would slowly disappear into the night the air would be filled with the sound of frogs calling out to each other. A choir of unique chirps, barks, clicks and croaks that broadcast advertisements of key information for each species. Males call out marking their territory, alerting each other of danger and most predominantly for mating purposes. Extra frisky frogs will make their calls during the day too. The louder and stronger the call, the more females it attracts. In certain species of frogs, the female calls out as well forming a duet which also helps the mating pair find each other in the vastness of night. Quite the romantic courtship if you ask me. For many others and I where we live, the songs of frogs have always been associated with the warming temperatures of spring and the promise of summer heat accompanied by all the exciting feelings that brings to life.

Once I woke up early in the morning during my summer holiday or on the weekends during school, the very first thing I thought about was returning to the area I was the day before catching frogs. I would barely eat my breakfast. I was so excited to get out the door into the Spring or Summer air and begin my quest to find the best spot along the ditches that were like marshes, by where I lived to catch frogs. I would usually bring an old empty ice cream pail and the lid would have many holes poked in it for proper oxygen flow. In which I would scoop up some of the dirty swampy water, add some little water plants and a branch or stick to recreate those cute little froggies' natural habitat. I did this so when I did catch frogs, I put them into the pail and they would feel at home, relaxed, and not threatened in a somewhat familiar environment. I would never ever hurt the frogs that I caught. I loved to study them. I would draw them, name them, talk to them. I would usually always release them at the end of the day, exactly where I caught them. However, there were a few sleepover nights occasionally, where I would keep them outside in the pail overnight. Then returning them first thing the next morning. I snuck them inside a few times as well. Most summer days I would be out there all by myself. The ditches along the perimeter Highway close to where I lived were endless and abundant at that time. They would stretch for as you could see. It was more like a marsh. At their widest point they were approximately thirty feet across and about five to six feet deep at some points, but most were about two to three feet deep. The moats were beautifully decorated with all types of flowers, bulrushes, tall grasses, and stunning water plants. At some points these creeks flooded, and small swampy pools were left behind in lower ground. These would make excellent habitats for frogs.

To become successful at catching frogs, one must master the art of stealth, patience, and observation. Using your ears to locate a frog by listening to its call helps with locating its proximity. Spotting frogs before it's too late to catch them is the trick of the trade. When a frog is spotted the frogger must remain absolutely motionless for a moment to allow the frog to reset its defensive mindset and then ever so slowly begin to position themselves to catch it. Relaxed and careful movements are crucial. Using an open hand, sweeping the frog up or palming it on the ground ensures that the frog will not be injured, which is critical when frogging. Sometimes by luck when you're walking alongside the creek you will startle a frog or two causing them to jump out and then you can catch them. Others, you would see floating in the water beside small lily pads, sometimes you would see them sitting on logs or rocks sunning themselves for energy. A homemade net would be a very useful tool for the safe capture of the frogs, especially those that were submerged in the water. I used an old wooden hockey stick with a butterfly net attached to it. This provided me with a good extension and was able to net frogs swimming as they swam away. A good frogger had to make sacrifices. Rubber boots were the best choice to wear but were uncomfortable and hot in the summer heat. They did keep your feet dry but impeded agility. Blisters from rubbing on the back of the heel was a common ailment from rubber boots. A pair of old running shoes usually were the preferred apparel. "Booters" were a common hazardous penalty while frog hunting. An uncertain step on the wrong compromised edge would cause your foot to become submerged in water and mud up to your ankles or even higher. Sometimes causing a fall into the creek. If you were out with some friends catching frogs and you got stuck in the mud with a booter it was fair game to throw mud balls at them to make them topple over into the water. As they say, "Without risk there is no reward."

It was imperative that I appreciated and studied every single species of frog that inhabited my demographic. It was key to have familiarity in each species' habits. Although, every single time I went out to catch frogs I fantasized that I would discover new species. Perhaps a prehistoric living fossil never seen before. What if I was the one that found a new species of amphibian or reptile thought to be long extinct. I imagined seeing alligators, crocodiles, and caimans in the water where I was frogging even though I knew that these large, beautiful reptiles lived far south from me. The four most common frogs that I would catch in order of most often caught were as follows:

The Northern Leopard Frog. A large frog. Its coloration could be bright or dark green or brown with large lightly etched dark spots all over its back and a white belly. They get their name from the Leopard like spot patterns. These frogs grow pretty big, up to a ten-centimeter body length but most are usually between five and eight centimeters on average. The Leopard Frog is an extraordinary jumper. In fact, their legs are longer than their body. This enables a Leopard Frog to leap thirteen times its own body length! Tricky when attempting to catch these lovely long jumpers! They have large, webbed feet which make them a commanding swimmer as well. They could be found on the edge of the water, in the water and the grasslands around it. These frogs will venture far from water making their way into forests and wooded areas on occasion. Female Leopard frogs can lay as many as five thousand eggs in a large jelly-like clutch attached to floating vegetation or branches in the early spring. The eggs hatch usually in about a week. Tadpoles will turn into froglets over roughly two months. I would always love catching tadpoles in a jar in their various stages of growth into becoming a full-grown frog. This species spends the winter hibernating underwater. Northern Leopard frogs can breathe through their skin. Finding a water source that has acceptable amounts of dissolved oxygen and will not freeze all the way to the bottom. This aids in oxygen and carbon passing through the frog's skin by diffusion. The frog will remain as motionless as possible at the bottom of the frozen pond, sometimes partially burying itself in mud leaving their backs exposed to breathe as well as prevent a hungry predator looking for a tasty snack. An evolutionary underwater breathing adaptation. On a warm sunny day, I would catch at least a dozen or so of these elusive and entertaining frogs every hunt.

Next up is the Wood Frog. A moderate sized frog that may be reddish, tan, or dark brown with a little bit of a black mask under its eyes, with a light line down the middle of its back. Their bellies are a creamy white and their toes are not fully webbed. On a good late spring/early summer day, I would usually catch about a half dozen of this species easily. Wood Frogs look like fallen leaves in their colorations making them masters of camouflage in their environment. I would find them during the day under rotting logs or rocks along the creeks or at the base of the surrounding woods. These frogs freeze sixty five percent solid during the winter underneath the woodland floor of leaves and fallen timber. They can freeze and thaw with their environmental conditions. As temperatures drop around minus five, ice crystals in the frog's skin, their liver produces heavy amounts of glucose that helps fill the emptied cells maintaining their structure. These frogs have special proteins in their blood that freeze quickly and form ice which in turn sucks out most of the water from the cells. Meaning that the frogs' shrunken cells are full of sugar which prevents freezing to death. The frog stops breathing, its heart stops beating and is in a state of suspended animation. It would appear to be dead, but when temperatures rise the ice in the body melts and the cells fill up with water, their hearts start to beat again.

They thaw, wake up and hop away towards the nearest water source to begin mating as early as late March. They will breed in creeks, ponds, marshes while the snow is still melting. Quite the remarkable environmentally amphibious adaptation in my opinion, amphibious antifreeze.

The next two species of frogs are classified as tree frogs. Both are very similar in size and habitat.

The spring peeper is a typical tree frog, small with large toe pads for climbing vegetation and varying skin color from tan, green, grey, a dull yellow and are easily distinguished from other tree frogs by a dark X on their back. They prefer the comfort of lower bushes or thick grass. The breeding call of the Spring Peeper is one of the earliest and loudest heard in the beginning of spring. These frogs reach no larger than three centimeters in length but they're breeding call can be heard over half a kilometer away. Their call is a single high-pitched peep repeated and can be deafening or exhilarating depending on proximity to the source. Once emerged from freezing over the winter, mating and breeding begins. The female Spring Peepers lay their eggs singularly along the bottom of ponds, swamps, and creeks.

The Boreal Chorus frog is another small smooth skin tree frog reaching a maximum length of four centimeters The color varies from green to Grey to Brown. There is a darker stripe through the eye and a white stripe along its upper lip. This one is recognizable because it has three distinguished dark stripes down its back. The Boreal Chorus Frog is the earliest mating call heard in spring. Boreal means "Northern" and a Chorus is a group of singers. This is how it has earned its namesake being a northern frog that sings love songs together in chorus into the night. The mating call sounds just like if you were to run your fingernail down the teeth of a plastic comb. These little frogs are the most common in population but still tricky to find and catch due to their small size and camouflage. These little cuties freeze every winter as well.

Both of these small tree frogs could be found anywhere from the brushing vegetation and bulrushes along the creek, or in the grasses along the water as well in the water too. The cutest of the frogs I would routinely catch and often the tamest. Sometimes as small as my thumbnail, these little tree frogs would perch on my finger and stay rested there absorbing my body warmth calmly observing me while I observed them.

There are other species that I caught that were not as abundant as the main four that I often encountered such as the Cope's Grey Tree Frog and the Gray Treefrog. These medium sized Tree Frogs that have a plump belly and long acrobatic legs with large suction cup like toe pads for climbing trees and branches. These were my absolute favorites to catch! Identical in appearance but separated by two chromosomes. The Cope's Gray has two sets of chromosomes whereas the Gray has four sets of chromosomes. Individuals are shades of brown, grey or green. They can change their coloration based on the temperature and lighting conditions in their environment making them true masters of camouflage. Becoming bright green to blend in on a large leaf or dark grey to match the tree bark of the branch it would be resting on. They have distinguishable bright yellow groins and inner thighs. I would on exceedingly rare occasions find these magnificent beauties resting in or around hollows in trees during the day. They spend much of their time in the forest canopy. The only way to tell the two species apart is by their breeding calls. One being higher pitched and more rapid than the other. Both are a medium sized frog growing to six centimeters and have bumpy skin texture resembling moss in appearance which helps camouflage in the trees in which they dwell. During the freezing winter months these tree frogs like the Wood Frog, Spring Peeper and Boreal Chorus Frog would hibernate in suspended animation under the forest floor. I only found them in the wooded areas that lined the creeks and ponds as the sun was setting and it was getting dark out. If I was lucky enough to be out at a lake or camping in the wilderness, I would find these tree frogs near a light source as they hunted for insects in the night. These, as most frogs, hunt nocturnally. I often got in trouble for not coming home when I was supposed to. Staying out way past my curfew, but it was worth every second of trouble I got into.

Then also there are toads. Often on the trails back when I was heading home, I would come across different species of toads slowly hopping across or along the pathway. Different from frogs because their skin is dry and bumpy and not silky and smooth like most frog's skin. Toads also don't need a direct water source to survive even though they are amphibians. Chubby and cumbersome in appearance making them extra cute, toads were usually an easy catch. I always thought they looked like they had a mischievous sense of humor by the look on their faces. Perhaps it was the way their mouth was configured. They have warts on their back and possess hard pads on their hind feet, like mini shovels, to aid in digging their way down in loose soil or in abandoned animal burrows below the frost line to survive the winter. Toads can excrete a foul-tasting liquid when attacked by a predator to protect its survival. Most animals will leave the toads alone due to this defensive mechanism. Snakes and birds are the primary predators of toads. Many times, I caught different toads and they would just calmly croak as they were handled. Sitting comfortably in the palm of my hand for long durations. To clear up the totally falsified myth that touching frogs or toads will give you warts, one must first understand that these amphibians do not possess any glands that produce any secretion that can cause warts. Although Toads may possess warts on their skin, they are completely different in composition from those that a human may encounter. Warts are caused by viruses in humans. Go wash your hands.

When I look back on my childhood and even into my teen years when I was catching frogs, I felt free. I felt like I belonged there. It became like a sanctuary, or one might say an escape for me. I would stay out as long as I could in the summer sun or even if it was raining. It didn't matter in the spring if it'd be cool in the fall or could be whatever I would still be out there from early in the morning, maybe come home for lunch. I would come in for supper powering through the meal and then I try to be back out to whatever time I was allowed out until. I hated being at home. There was an abundance of awful things going on at that time in my life. I felt like no one could hurt me when I was out there catching frogs. My favorite times were when I would catch a frog and hold it gently in my hand, looking into its eyes. I would slowly open my hand and sometimes the frog would immediately jump away, but other times the frog would stay in the palm of my hand for a while, looking right back at me. I felt connected to that frog. Connected to the innocence of mutual trust inside nature. A connection I did not feel with people. I often would talk to the frogs about what was happening at home. I would ask them questions -why were these things happening to me? Why were people hurting me so bad? Why didn't anyone like me?

I was getting severely bullied by older kids in my neighborhood. The kids knew how to set me off and then would take turns trying to beat me up. Chase me and when they caught me would call me retard and hold my eyes wide open and take turns spitting in my eyes. Flipping my eyelids inside out.

The worst time I remember was when I was alone walking home from catching frogs alongside the creek. It was starting to get dark out. Up ahead were a group of teens from the high school drinking alcohol and smoking cigarettes along the path home. I had a few frogs left in my pail as I was about to return them to where I caught them closer to home. One of the older boys started walking towards me saying "hey retard boy. What's in the bucket?" I knew things were about to get ugly so I took off running as fast as I could, but they caught up to me and kicked my legs out from under me. I crashed hard into the ground. One of the bigger boys sat on top of me, holding me down. I could smell the potency of alcohol on his breath as he said, "don't ever make me run again, retard boy" and proceeded to punch me in the back of my head. The others opened up the bucket and started laughing saying "aww are these your little friends? They probably think you are a stupid retard like everybody else does". He then poured out the remaining frogs onto the pathway floor and started to stomp and kill my frogs. I tried so hard to get free but the kid on top of me was way bigger and stronger than I was. He slapped me repeatedly in the face telling me to shut up and then punched me in the stomach so hard I could not breathe for a few seconds. When I caught my breath, I started screaming to "stop hurting the frogs, they did nothing wrong to you!" They all laughed at me and said "now you have no friends, they are all dead" as he stomped on the last frog that was alive. I was so mad, heartbroken. I was screaming for help and started crying because I couldn't believe anyone would be so mean and kill those frogs like that. Then their focus turned to me. The whole group was very drunk. There were five of them. They were making comments about me being a little cry baby and that they were going to give me something to cry about. One of the boys grabbed a hold of my legs while the other one was still holding me down. A third teenager walked up and said he had to take a piss really bad and was going to piss on my face to wash my cry baby tears away. I remember he was wearing white runners that were stained from mud. His jeans stained from the grease of his bicycle chain. I closed my eyes and held my breath as he started urinating on my face, trying my hardest to move my face out of the way. All I could hear was their laughter. I tried to bite the leg of the kid that was standing over me. That's when another boy kicked me in the testicles so hard, I immediately opened my eyes and my mouth to scream in pain. They picked me up by my arms and legs and swung me back and forth like a swing launching me into the water. It was only about a foot deep where I landed. I was soaking wet, muddy, in so much pain, humiliated and disgraced. All I could think about as I crawled out of the water was about the frogs that they killed. I was so irate and heartbroken. I remember at that moment I wished I had superpowers like superhuman strength so I could grab them and pick them up, smashing them into the ground, ripping them in half and throwing their dead bodies far off into the horizon. As a small rock hit me on the side of the head and cut me open, the impact brought me back to reality. They started throwing more rocks at me as I ran away as fast as I could. I never looked back, I just kept running and running. When I got home, I was still drenched, and I was late. My dad asked why I was soaking wet and covered in mud and what happened to the side of my head. I told him that I fell into the creek, but I was fine. He said to me "you don't look fine to me, son." I wanted to tell him everything, but I just kept it inside. Then he told me to go rinse myself and my shoes off with the hose outside. To this very day, I can still remember the rancid taste of urine in my mouth and how bad it stung and burnt in my eyes. I was eight years old.

Years later, I would turn what I learnt from my frog hunting skills into becoming very successful at people hunting. I made sure that every one of those boys who were now men, remembered exactly what they did that day. On behalf of the frogs, of course. Wink, wink. Ribbit, ribbit.

More significantly, catching frogs was the means of distracting myself from what was happening at home when I was young. As I mentioned, once I was out of the house and out there in nature with my amphibious friends, I felt free. Where I belonged. I had a purpose. My imagination could uninterruptedly run wild. It was uncontainable and limitless. I suppose it was a form of meditation. Moments that became hours, sitting there listening to the wind and how it caressed the leaves and tall grasses around me. Birds sang to each other in symphonic frequencies. The rest of the world held still and faded away. It was like it did not even exist. It was just me and nature.

There was a woman in my father's life that came along at the same time as the bullying, a while after he and my mother had divorced. In the beginning of their relationship, she seemed ok, but I always had feelings of intuitive apprehension around her. Once she moved in with us, from the very start, when my father was not around, she made it very clear she did not want me there. At first, she would act nice and sweet when my dad and sister were present. When I was alone with her is when she began to do horrible things to me. I was having a lot of difficulties at school with comprehension and learning. Had issues with my behavior. A kind way to say I was delayed compared to the other kids in my class. I remember the first time she locked me in a closet and told me that I was a retard and that my dad hates me and was embarrassed to be my father. That he wished I was dead. This would become a very common ritual for her. The more time she spent with my dad the worse her behavior towards me increased. She would choke me; she would kick my testicles and grab my penis and squeeze as hard as she could until I cried or passed out in pain. One time she took a lighter and burnt the base of my penis because I tracked some mud onto the carpet by the front door when I had returned from catching frogs. She would lock me in my room regularly, abuse me and tell me she would kill me and my sister if I ever said anything to my dad. She told me that she wanted to burn me alive because that is what I deserved. I reminded her of my mother and that my father once was with her. Beyond jealousy, it was pathological and psychotic. She sprayed cleaning products in my eyes and said things like oh look at the little retard crying. She would get on top of me, choking me to near unconsciousness, a few times she put me out. She went through my father's photo album and destroyed every picture of me from when I was a baby up to the current age I was then. Any of the remaining pictures of my dad and I together, she took the liberty to cut me out of the picture completely. She even cut out pictures of herself and then proceeded to tape them into the original where I used to be. I tried telling my dad, but I was terrified to tell him everything because she told me she would kill my sister and I if I ever said anything.

It had gotten so bad at one point that I started learning how to tie knots, so I could hang myself. I was in Cub Scouts and had a booklet on knots. A slip knot was the preferred knot to get the jo done. I hated being alive. I hid it all the time, pretending like I was fine. I hated that too. The only time I was fine was when I was catching frogs, playing outside with my friends or if I was alone with my dad, at my grandparents' house, or visiting my mom. My dad had some yellow rope in the storage closet by his tools in our townhouse that I used. I waited until everyone had gone to bed. At first, I tried to hang myself on my bunk bed, but it wasn't quite high enough. I moved my efforts to the closet, and I tied myself up on the wooden rod that goes across the closet to hang clothes on. I tried to hang myself there. I wrapped the rope multiple times around the wooden rod, standing on a stepping stool as I secured the noose around my neck. I anticipated a swift end to my pain. When I kicked out the stool, I remember feeling the force of my weight drop causing extreme pressure around my neck with the noose tightening instantly. I reached up with my arms and held onto the rope around my neck. I uncontrollably kicked my legs out frantically as I was going out of consciousness and that caused one of the plastic brackets on the wall that held the wooden pole in place to break. I fell to the ground and desperately freed myself from the noose around my neck and took a huge gulp of air. I lied there crying in shame for about half an hour. I was nine years old and in grade four.

As time went on so that the abuse and the torture continued with me, but a lot of her psychotic behavior began to surface in front of my father and my sister. She began lashing out at my dad verbally and physically. She was mean to my sister as well, but luckily for her, she lived with my mom and only came over on the weekends. My sister and I would talk about how scared we were of her to each other secretly in fear of her finding out. Finally, after things got crazy between her and my pops, he finally began to understand the things my sister and I were telling him about her. She went psychotic when they broke up. Threatening to kill herself. To kill my father. Well as a woman of her word, she lived up to her promise as she did try to kill me. A few months later, my sister and I were walking home together from playing in the field nearby. It was a hot and sunny Saturday afternoon. As we approached the side-by-side house we relocated to, I noticed that the aluminum screen door was left open. This was odd because anytime I left that door the least bit open by accident, my dad always had something to say about it. Usually pertaining to allowing all the mosquitoes, flies, and wasps in the world to fly inside the house. My sister who was younger than me by two years, was walking in front of me into the house and I was a couple steps behind her. Suddenly and unexpectedly, from around the corner behind a wall, that crazed woman jumped out and she was in possession of a knife as long as her forearm. It was like one of those big sharp kitchen knives. Like the ones used to carve turkeys. We were both shockingly terrified. The look in her eyes was sinister and maniacal. I grabbed my little sister and put her behind me so she would be safe, stretching my arms out to the sides to block her advance from any angle. I knew she was there to kill me, she hated me and wanted me dead. She had blamed me for everything and now it was time for her revenge. Just as she started to lunge towards me with the knife and extended her arm in an overhead stabbing motion targeting my chest, my father came running out of another room, grabbed her, and tackled her into a nearby wall. He started screaming at my sister and I to get out of the house. She was trying to stab him in the chest and neck. They went up and down the stairs, fighting. She was screaming that she wanted to kill him and then herself. After what seemed like hours but, within seconds my dad had pinned her to the ground and got the knife away from her. I remember him looking at us with panic and horror in his eyes. It was the first time that I had ever seen my dad cry. I finally felt like that nightmare was over.

I guess this is why I put so much energy into learning all the habits. The details. While studying the movements of frogs, I found the more time I dedicated to studying how to catch frogs, I would remain happy and be at peace. It was almost an obsession catching those cute little bulgy eyed frogs. I would name every single one of them that I caught because it made the connection more significant and personal. I wanted to draw and sketch them later at night when I was afraid to go to bed, which was every night. I would be trapped awake all night with my overthinking brain spinning funnels of out-of-control thoughts. Focusing on each of their unique details while drawing then eased my mind to sleep. The activity of catching frogs was a survival tactic that I was unaware of at that time. As I look back on that particular part of my life, I've come to realize that without those frogs and my attachment to them, I may not be here today. It was such an alluring and educational distraction. Teaching me about myself and life. Yes, there were horrible experiences associated with catching frogs like the bullying and the psychological trauma I was exposed to through the abuse by that woman, however the activity of catching frogs remains as an uplifting and enriching experience in my life today. It helped me to not feel as alone or hurt. My mind was so consumed with the constant stimulus of the natural environment and activities that I could separate myself from the reality of my life. Fear no longer made the rules when it came to my decisions. Although I had been previously physically and emotionally hurt, I would not mentally break. While I was fixated on catching frogs, I did not need anyone to hold my hand. Tell me that it was ok. I adapted quickly through trial and error. Failure was fun and I looked forward to it. Failure just meant a new opportunity to get back out there and work on improving the precision of my techniques. Throughout all the experiences, good or bad, the dynamics never really changed as long as I had something sacred to hold on to like frog hunting. All the involved circumstances of the experiences served as a lesson.

To this day I will take any opportunity to catch frogs. passing on my knowledge as a master of the craft to any open mind possible. Educating people on the importance that frogs play in our ecosystems and that they are in fact a determining staple in the health of those ecosystems. Regardless of age, or where you live from the Arctic to the Sahara, frogs are abundant everywhere and waiting to be found. It also doesn't matter how old you are because I believe you're never too old to have fun. Take yourself, or if you have children on a nice nature discovery day. Go catch frogs together as a family or a group, or by yourself. Instill a love of the natural world while it is still possible. I can guarantee you that it would be an amazing and comical time that might just provide some fun filled stories to share. Providing an opportunity to even learn something about yourself in the process as well. I suppose it's also safe to say that as adults if we were to embrace more things that we loved like when we were kids, perhaps we wouldn't be so bitter and unhappy. I'm not sure who made the rules that we must stop being a kid just because we get older. Of course, there are more responsibilities as adults. Imagine doing things you loved in the time between. A child-like approach to challenge could change everything in life, in my opinion. It would certainly brighten up the dull and tarnished times of just sitting around watching television or on the computer, complaining about the same thing every day like a broken record. Children rarely make excuses not to have fun. Show your kids or loved ones what you loved doing when you were a kid. Do things that you loved when you were a kid with your children, family, and your friends. When we see others doing something with passion and love it is intoxicatingly contagious. If you do not have kids, then do It for yourself. Re-open the mind to imagination. Hop back on that skateboard. Skip rope. Ride bicycles. Smell flowers. Watch your favorite childhood movie. Hike the mountain. Fill your pockets with shells and rocks. Go on adventures. Bust out that air guitar and rock out. Get outside and explore this vibrant ever-changing painting of biodiversity that is of our world. The fear of what everyone else would think if we did something fun was non-existent as a child. Connect with that and catch frogs or whatever it was for you as a child, every day. We can look for the bad or good in anything. What we choose is our responsibility to ourselves, however it does impact ripples in the ponds of life. We can choose to be the victim, or we can choose to be the reason the victimization ends. Either way, it will influence the people around you. Unfulfilling or fulfilling, misery or happiness. Becoming inspirational by encouraging everyone by marching to the beat of your own drums as you dance like a fool without fear or the need for validation. I provided the timbers that steadily coaxed the fires of my own depression until I was able to understand how I chose to see things could change the outcome of what happened in my past. I chose to see like a child again. This would gently help extinguish the slow burn of the side effects of my mental illness as I became able to opt for more positive perspectives over dismal perceptions of myself and my past experiences.

On every single trip I have taken in this world, I have taken with me my love for catching frogs and discovered new worlds full of excitement every time. The simple act of just doing something that I have loved doing since I was a kid has inspired so many other people to join me in my quest to catch frogs. People of all kinds and from places all around the world have told me how much they loved catching frogs when they were young. I would always smile and say to them that it looks like you still love it today. As my good friend Kermit, the Frog once said "Take a look above you, discover the view. If you haven't noticed, please do."

CHAPTER 5

CAVIA PORCELLUS

If you cage the beast, the beast will get angry.
Wolverine

From a very young age I had exhibited some unconventional behaviors and had difficulty learning like the other kids my age. I was always fun loving and liked to play with other kids. Very quirky and peculiar. I began my role as a comedian/class clown around nine years old in Grade Four. It was my way of forgetting about all the hell I was going through at the time. My audience were the kids in my class and not so much my teachers. My stage was my classroom. I would do anything to get my classmates laughing uncontrollably, even if it meant the small sacrifice of a trip to the principal's office where I had become a regular visitor. The principal at my school always stunk of whiskey. His nose was swollen with red and purple broken blood capillaries from all the alcohol he consumed. I knew this because he enjoyed screaming at me up close and personal. He also liked to punish me by bending me over his desk, pulling my pants down and smacking my bare ass relentlessly. Until he got tired. He would be wheezing and yell at me that "boys like you are going straight to hell!"" I would always laugh when he said that to me. The joke was on him, I was already there.

I began to have violent outbursts if I felt like someone was making fun or mocking me. I kind of felt like the hulk. I would explode with anger and do the most impulsive and craziest things. Afterwards, once I began calming down, I would feel really bad about what I did. Remorseful. I didn't understand why I behaved this way. It was an uncontrollable reaction. With no solution in sight. Sadly, I never turned green or became a hulking giant to my dismay.

I was severely bullied for the majority of early elementary school years. Dispassionately always being the new kid at school made me a sitting duck. Many of the kids at school knew how to trigger me to get upset so they could sit back and watch the freakshow. I was called a retard often because I was having difficulty learning like the other kids in my classes. I was relentlessly picked on because I was so small and skinny compared to the other kids my age. I was an easy target to manipulate because I wanted to fit in with the other kids so badly and I found myself falling victim to many set ups that would humiliate me in my endless pursuit of acceptance of the other kids. I would scream and swear, throw things like books, staplers, scissors, chairs, and eventually desks at other students and my teachers as this continued as I grew older. Sometimes, I would run away for the day and not return to school. Other times I wouldn't return until later in the night. There was a small department store a few blocks away from my school. I would go there and steal things like toys, books, and pornographic magazines. I would also stop in at the convenience store and fill my pockets with all my favorite chocolate bars and candies. I got caught by the police sometimes. They would give me a long boring lecture and then return me to my school if it was during school hours or my home if later in the day. Neither one was an enjoyable experience to say the least.

During this same time, I was going through horrific abuse from my dad's girlfriend. Making going home a deterring encumbrance. I would often get in trouble because I would wander around for hours after school and come home late at night

It was fair to say that all the trauma that I had been through was radically surfacing in my behaviors. My outbursts were becoming more uncontrollable by the day. I hid behind anger and wore it like a mask. I had begun my dual life in these very moments. Making everyone else laugh and feel happy was my priority while simultaneously I was self-deconstructing inside. Unravelling.

I started over again at another school. Over the next two school years, my eruptions were getting more powerful, more frequent and lasting longer. I was having trouble containing myself. My standup comedy and class clowning was beginning to share the spotlight with surges of violent behavior and self-harm. From Kindergarten to Grade six, I went to five different elementary schools. So, I had no choice but to learn how to become a chameleon. Reinventing myself while meeting all new kids in a new classroom at that age was terrifying. I had to do it over and over.

I started lying compulsively to everyone I met. Trying to make myself seem more interesting, so I could fit in. A spectacular illusion created by clever story telling accompanied by my wild imagination. I was starting to believe my own lies. Then they became my truths. Between creating fantasy worlds where I wished I lived, to the lies I would tell, I was very, very lost. I always felt as though I was never good enough for people to like me. But every chance I got, I still tried to make everyone laugh. I tried to make them happy. My perception of my young self was clearly distorted.

I started at a new school in grade five. This was the fifth school I had attended already. My dad had stopped drinking and partying, got clean and sober and moved in with an amazing new woman who inspired him to do so. She was very kind, understanding and compassionate with him and I. The outright opposite of what I had previously been exposed to. She would marry my father and change both our lives for the better. We had moved again. This time we were in the same area of a neighborhood, but I had to change schools. I actually ended up liking this school and made some good friends. A few lifelong friends. We played Dungeons and Dragons often. They would take the time to teach me how to play because I could not comprehend it until they showed me. Of course, they would frequently coach me into a game ending move that they would laugh so hard at. It was funny. We also played outdoor sports like ice and street hockey. We played war in the woodlands surrounding our houses. Pairing up in teams of soldiers. We would hide in the trees and in the brushland, attempting to "kill" the other team. We were also ninjaing as well at nighttime. We made homemade ninja weapons and used Black Widow Slingshots. Masters of invisibility or so we thought until we would get caught by the police sneaking around the neighborhood late at night. A few years later we would build a halfpipe ramp in one of the backyards and we rode BMX 's and skateboards. Let the good times roll.

Although, being new there would normally be challenging, my teacher Mr. B made the assimilation easily adaptable and enjoyable. I would assemble a good core group of friends for the first time, my grades improved somewhat, my home was for the first time that I could remember had become peaceful. Looking back, I wasn't sure I knew how to enjoy that as it was so foreign to me.

Although I could never remain focused for long, and was distracted by everything, ticking clocks on the wall above the chalkboard, someone else talking, or just wandering off in my mind and feeling like the walls were closing in on me constantly. I found a new passion. A beautiful distraction. I loved drawing and I loved comic books. My favorites were the X-Men. Mutants that through genetic mutation had gained superpowers. Many of them were outcasts and did not belong anywhere, alienated because of their abilities. Often exiled from their own family because they were different. Some of them went through life altering adversity that triggered their mutation. Out of the vast universe of the X-Men, Wolverine was my undeniable favorite. Born on Canadian soil, somewhere near Cold Lake, Alberta, James "Logan" Howlett would become the Wolverine. A tortured soul who often tiptoed down the line of being a hero or an anti-hero. Through a brain damaging incident, Wolverine could not remember most of the details of his previous life and was lost inside himself endlessly trying to find out who he was. Where he belonged. He was a super soldier. His character was violent and angry and, in some situations, compassionate but always protecting the ones closest to him. His mutant ability was a constant healing factor of his own body, never aging, or getting sick and any wounds he suffered would heal themselves instantly. He had heightened animal-like keen senses and was a savage warrior. Originally, he had three bone-like claws that came out of his knuckles on each hand. Later due to his ability to heal he became a candidate for an experimental military operation that would lace his skeleton with an alien metal that was indestructible called adamantium. His retractable claws became long metal blades capable of cutting through anything which was accompanied by superhuman strength and other physical capabilities. Becoming a super soldier. Wolverine would defy the military powers trying to control him to be a weapon and escape, eventually join the X-Men. A team of mutants that provided hope and fought evil for both normal people and mutants alike.

I began learning how to draw comic book-like characters. Continually sketching all day and night. Creating my own universe of characters. I integrated new worlds in new galaxies. I would draw my future-self as a muscular barbaric loner, yielding a razor-sharp battle axe in one hand and in the other hand I had the power to absorb energy and manipulate it into a cosmic burst of solar energy. Superhuman intelligence mixed with superhuman strength made my character a worthy adversary in any arena of battle. Driven with an undying thirst for blood and vengeance. In my superhero world, I was an anti-hero that brought balance to justice, but often crossed the line in doing so. My character's brooding nature was violent and sought-after redemption. This helped me to distract myself from reality.

My homeroom teacher Mr. B. was an extraordinary man. Tall, thin but athletic build, silver hair and glasses. He was incredibly charismatic, and his smile and laughter were always contagious. He loved to run, and I joined his running club. We would meet an hour before school started and jog through the neighborhood. I loved being a part of it. Teaching us the importance of physical exercise to start the day to set a positive mind and a sense of accomplishment. He was kind and compassionate towards me and all his students. Never once showing any form of frustration or anger in his classroom. He would take me aside if he saw that I was struggling and softly speak to me reminding me that it was okay if I did not understand the work in front of me and that he would help me. His patience was at a level I had never experienced. Everyday Mr. B made school amusing and enjoyable. Which helped his students to learn at a very rapid rate. He was not like most traditional teachers. In class we would put on plays about the books we were reading. He was an accomplished musician and would bust out his acoustic guitar and play music that we would creatively shape the lyrics to, bluegrass songs that he would sing to us and then ask the class for their interpretation of it. He taught the class about animals through catchy songs we would all sing along together to. Mr. B always smiled in a way you felt it in your heart. His sense of humor was warm and inviting. My outbursts had become few and far between in his classroom. Mr. B had a magical way of keeping me calm and focused. He had a strong relationship with me. Always making the effort to understand what was bothering me without judgment. Keeping myself and the other kids engaged through lots of interactive educational activities. Blossoming the minds of all the kids he entertained while educating them. Experiential learning at its finest.

While we were running together in the mornings before school, Mr. B would ask me all kinds of questions about my dreams, my hopes, what I wanted to be when I grew up. I didn't really have any answers for him. One day after we had finished our run, we had been talking in depth about what he saw as my potential. He looked at me kindly and said "Jason, I think you are incredible. I believe that if you could focus all your energy into a positive force, you could become anything you want, I think you could change the world Jason, I truly do." I have never forgotten those words throughout my lifetime.

I would bump into Mr. B from time to time and he would always ask me how my dad was doing and follow up with how I was doing as well. Later in life I found out that Mr. B was nominated for a Juno Award in 2002 "Call of The Wild" for best children's recording in Canada. He routinely performed at The Winnipeg Folk Festival, where he was described as one of Canada's most treasured performers and musical educators. So, two decades later, I went to go see him perform and tell him thank you for all he did to help me. The Winnipeg Folk Festival is a nonprofit charitable organization. Hosting a tremendous outdoor annual summer festival featuring musicians and artists from all over the world, as well as many local artists. With as many as seventy thousand people attending the festival making it one of the most premier outdoor concerts in North America. From my experience I found it to be a very open and free love spirited event. All walks of life enjoy the energy together. The day I attended to see Mr. B perform, was a scorching hot July day in the prairies. I was very excited to see him and tell him how much he had positively influenced my mind. At the same time years of suppressed pain and guilt that I felt from letting him down when I had acted out during school were beginning to swell tears in my eyes. The last time I had seen Mr. B was in my late teens so twenty years later I looked a little different than what he remembered me as, I'm sure. To paint the picture accurately, I had gained seventy pounds of muscle, much of my upper body covered in tattoos, and my face looked like carved rock. I had no shirt on, for the people who know me, this will come as no surprise. The last time he saw me, I was a scrawny little boy. I entered the massive tent in which Mr. B was performing. I could hear his invigorating and animated voice immediately giving me goosebumps. Inside the tent were hundreds of people, families, kids. The stage was wrapped with so many kids singing and laughing, some dancing, while others watching. There I stood. Frozen in between my childhood and the present. I was overtaken by a landslide of emotion. Reverting to so many feelings of shame that I felt because I could not control myself the way I wanted to back then. All I could do was stand there and cry. As a moment passed and I regained a fraction of my composure I started waving at him like an excited child trying to get his attention in class. On stage with him was his lifelong love who was also one of my teachers at the same time as him back in the eighties. She was as beautiful as I remembered, I could hear her sweet soft voice inside my head. She was interacting with the children during the songs he sang. When Mr. B finally got a glance of me, his facial expression changed for a brief second to one of slight concern. From his perspective there was a large muscular tattooed man standing in the middle of his audience of children with his shirt off balling and waving at him. After a second or two he smiled back at me and carried on with his performance. As intimidating as I looked to most people generally, the children and their families seemed nonjudgmental or threatened as I had a mental breakdown right there in front of them, while children's songs were being sung and children and their parents danced around me. What a sight that must have been.

After the performance Mr. B. came out and talked to me. He didn't recognize me at first glance, but I could see the wheels of memory turning in his eyes. His face lit up and he said "Jason McLean!" and then I instantly burst into tears again, telling him I was sorry for all the times I was bad. That I didn't mean to be so much trouble. He cracked up laughing, stating that I wasn't that bad, and he was so happy to see me. He said I was one of his most interesting students. He asked how my dad was doing. We chatted for about ten minutes and by the end of our conversation I had the biggest smile upon my face. I was beaming. I told him that he had been one of the most influential people in my life and thanked him for that graciously.

Being in his presence whether back when I was a boy or when I was a grown man, his energy was infinitely contagious, leaving me always wanting to do my best and enjoying it while I did. His compassion and dedication to opening and enhancing minds through creative and interactive education were more effective than all the other teachers combined throughout all my years of schooling. In one school year, I learned and retained more information about the world, people, and myself than all other years combined of school. All because of one teacher's influence, kindness, understanding and acceptance. Be that teacher.

My violent episodes had slowed down somewhat for the first couple weeks of school in Grade six. I had a new homeroom teacher and a new class. All was going well until one morning during science class. My teacher had a habit of pointing out when I was wrong about something in front of my class. Which was humiliating and embarrassing. She seemed very bitter and unhappy on a consistent basis and was regularly very condescending. It was though she really hated her career choice, perhaps she had been calloused over the years and completely lost her love of teaching and influencing young minds. I know that I was a tough challenge as a student because most of my previous teachers made that very clear to me and my parents. This teacher was not set up with the proper tools to deal with me. Instead, she sent me to the principal's office every opportunity she could and made it very known that I was struggling to learn as fast as the other kids. That her recommendation was to hold me back a year. On that day, the class was learning about Snapping Turtles. A species I was very familiar with as I had tried to catch them unsuccessfully several times. My dad had sold encyclopedias door to door at one time. He had a set of them leftover and gave them to me, as well I had another set of encyclopedias on animals that I received as a Christmas gift. I would spend my free time memorizing everything. Drawing the animals. Understanding all their details and characteristics. My favored subject was the classification of the natural world. There are seven classifications which aid in understanding how all living organisms are related. To break it down, the model looks like this: Kingdom, Phylum, Class, Order, Family, Genus and Species. The snapping turtle's classification table was like this: Kingdom-Animals, Phylum-Chordata, Class-Reptilia, Order-Testudines, Family-Chelydridae, Genus-Chelydra and Species-C. Serpentina. These are Latin obviously. C. Serpentina means snake-like and is based on their very mobile head and neck and its ability to strike its prey. Through Taxonomy, which is the study of naming, defining, and classifying organisms based on shared characteristics/binomial nomenclature, two termed naming systems are basically the laws of the classification system. I spent many hours back then memorizing this as well as the Snapping turtle 's ecology, anatomy, habitat, its part in the food chain and behavior.

My teacher had written "facts" upon the chalkboard about Snapping Turtles. I was really excited we were learning about these turtles. However, there were two small discrepancies written on the board. In fact, they were incorrect. When she asked the class if there were any questions, I raised my hand. She rolled her eyes as she said "yes, Jason?" in a tone that was presumptuous. I said "there were two things on the board that were incorrect about snapping turtles. The first one she had written said that Snapping Turtles hibernate all winter and the second was that they laid 5-10 eggs. I explained that Snapping Turtles have been swimming under the ice for months into winter and are the only cold tolerant turtle. Not all did this but not all hibernated. Some remained active under the ice all winter. I also explained that hibernating Snapping Turtles do not breathe air for six months. That they had a unique way of respirating due to their hibernation site being completely covered by ice and snow. I then explained that Snapping Turtles lay 25-80 eggs in a clutch, usually in a sandy muddy area away from water, and that my dad and I had come across one of these nesting sites near a lake in Ontario. I was not looking to start a problem; I was so happy we were studying biology because finally I could express my love for nature and share what I knew with her and the class for the sole purpose of education and to be able speak with confidence for once because I was very familiar with this subject. I felt like a normal kid at that moment. I felt like what all the other kids got to feel like during class.

My teacher responded quickly and sharply stating that I was wrong, that I had no idea what I was talking about and then scorned me for interrupting her. I replied that I didn't interrupt her because she had asked if there were any questions. She argued with me on that too. Blood starts boiling. I told her that I read encyclopedias every night and that is where my information came from, and my dad was the one who found the nest and identified them as snapping turtle eggs because of how many and how big the eggs were. She snapped back saying that she could hardly believe that I spent any time reading because I never completed my assignments and that she had to correct constantly when I was asked to read out loud. She then added that my dad was wrong and did not know what he was talking about. Blood reaches boiling point. I told her that my dad would never ever tell me something that was not true. He would never lie to me. In front of my entire class, she told me that my dad had lied to me about this, not that he may have made a mistake, that he was lying. My dad was far from perfect and made many mistakes, but he was never a liar. She told me if I said another word I would be sent to the principal's office. Blood boils over. I was standing there breathing fire, I was so mad at her. Humiliated again and now she had insulted my dad. I picked up the stapler on my desk and screamed and threw it at her. It hit the wall beside her head. I then picked up my chair and threw it at her, this time I hit her on the side of her shoulder and arm with it. I flipped my desk over and stomped out of class punching the walls on the way out. Another teacher attempted to stop me in the hallway between classrooms, but I pushed my way through him. Out the door I went. I didn't go home. I walked to a forested area, where my friends and I would hide away from everyone and build forts out of branches. I was there for hours when one of my buddies rolled up on his BMX and told me that my dad was looking for me. He had been calling all my friends' houses trying to find me and driving around. Time to face the music kid. What an awful song it would turn out to be.

I was suspended for a week, had to write a "meaningful" apology letter to my teacher, finish all curriculum and assignments, and that I was being moved to a different class upon my return. My new teacher was a man, and my desk was going to be located outside the classroom in an office pod. Therefore, I would be alone and unable to disrupt my class ever again. Problem solved. Animal contained.

Upon my return, I was greeted by my principal who was a fair man. The vice principal, she was a very kind and strong woman, a guidance counselor, another kind woman who truly seemed like she wanted to help me and make a difference and finally a resource teacher who was going to help me with my schoolwork. They all spoke to me about the expectations, often interrupting each other. I don't remember too much of it, but I do remember how bright the lights were in that room and that the principal was tapping his foot repeatedly while clicking his pen. I was told to be a good boy in my new kennel. No barking or biting.

I didn't last very long in my new enclosure. I hated my cage. The fluorescent lights buzzed like an old loud refrigerator. I could not sit still. I felt like the walls were going to close in on me. The unbroken tick tock of the clock on the wall above me was like a constant drum beat from a marching band reverberating inside my head. Kids would walk by and laugh at me between classes. Some were sympathetic in their gestures. Sometimes I would pretend I was sleeping or dead on my desk to make them laugh harder. I would draw signs that said, "help me" or "call 911", anything to feel connected to the other kids through shared laughter. The odd cartoon penis drawing would usually get the best reactions of uncontrolled laughter from everyone as they walked by and on to their next classroom. Teachers were never a fan of that, never appreciating my artwork.

I was kindly allowed the luxury of participating in gym class and intramural sports during lunch hour. Everything was going somewhat according to the caged animal plan until one day during intramural sports we were playing a game of floor hockey. I was on a team of three playing against another team of three. On the other team was the biggest kid in our school. He was loud, boisterous, cocky and liked to pick on me. I was the smallest boy in my grade, the shortest and skinniest of them all. Because it was during lunch, other kids were allowed to sit in the stands and watch. On this day the second prettiest girl according to the rating system of my friends was sitting behind the net up in the stands. I thought she was the prettiest, for the record and I had a big crush on her. Game starts, evenly matched teams, a good element of competition. About five minutes into the game, I was on a breakaway and about to score in front of my crush. This was it. The Big moment. She would see my skills and immediately fall in love with me obviously and we would live happily ever after. As I wound up for the shot and my moment of glory was about to take place, the big kid on the other team threw his floor hockey stick across the gymnasium shellacked hardwood floor, it skipped across and just as I was connecting with the plastic puck, his stick became entangled between my feet, and I tripped while shooting. I hit the floor with a massive painful thud, I could hear everyone's laughter in slow motion. As I looked up at my crush, she was crying and holding her face. The floor hockey puck had hit her in the bottom of her eye socket and the bridge of her nose which was bleeding. She hurtfully screamed at me "why would you do that? What is wrong with you?!" My big moment was destroyed. I turned around to see that big fat kid was on his knees laughing at me hysterically. Everyone was laughing at me. Except her. I was humiliated, embarrassed, heartbroken, and ashamed. Then the switch flipped. Gasket blown. It was time to get even. I could feel the pain of every single time I had been made fun of, neglected, hurt, humiliated, embarrassed, and alienated. The next forty-five seconds would change the course of my life. I ran as fast as I could out of the gym while more kids heckled and mocked me as I passed by them, adding more fuel to the fire in my head. I ran down the halls to my bubble where my desk was located, I slid open the tote tray under my desk and grabbed a big pair of scissors and ran back to the gym like a flash of lightning. As I entered, most of the kids were talking and still laughing at my expense. As soon as I spotted him, I charged towards that big kid. He ruined my life, now it was my time to ruin his. I lunged at him and began to extend my arm holding the scissors to stab him in the chest. Halfway through the motion I was tackled like a linebacker blindsiding a quarterback. My gym teacher took me to the ground hard. He pinned me there and put his knee on my forearm causing me to release the scissors. He was shaking. He looked at me and asked in a frantically charged voice "Jason! What the hell are you doing!!!???" Over and over. I remember looking up at him and saying I was sorry. I instantly felt bad for what I did. A couple more teachers ran in and helped hold me down, even though I was not fighting to get free. They held me there until the police arrived.

My fate lay in the hands of the big boy's parents. The Police threatened to charge with attempted murder and told me all these horror stories of prison. "You know what happens to little boys like you in jail?" When I said I'm too young to go to jail, the cops stated that they would make an exception on my behalf. Outstanding police work. The parents decided not to press charges against me. My school had expelled me originally but made a proposition to my parents and I, which was that I could come back to school as long as I agreed to see a psychiatrist to prescribe medication after my diagnosis, meet with a guidance counselor, a social worker and a child psychologist two times every week and my desk would be now in the office, in the guidance counselor's lounge away from all the other students, I would not be allowed outside for recess or lunch, participate in any field trips, no gym class and I was to have an adult chaperone me to and from school. I would start at 9:15 am so I would not interact with the other children outside and leave at 3:45 pm for the same reason. I remember sitting there looking out the window when my dad turned to me with a downhearted look in his eyes and asked me a few questions about following all these guidelines. I just agreed robotically. The Guidance Counselor was wrapping everything up and asked if I had any questions. I asked if I could just go to jail instead? Not one adult in that room appreciated the humor in my request. Case closed.

As my meetings commenced with all my new friends, there was a common concern amongst them all. "What was wrong with me?" I was told that the only way they could help me was to find out all the things wrong with me. Sign me up! Let the healing begin.

My guidance counselor was a sweet and compassionate woman. She had my best interest in her heart. I could make her laugh all the time with a technique that I had mastered. She had to escort me to the washroom anytime I needed to go. She would stand outside the door and wait for me. I then would proceed to make the loudest fart noises I possibly could with my mouth and my hands held around my mouth to amplify the thunderous onslaught of long fart noises and then make comments about how I couldn't stop farting as loud as I could. She would crack up laughing and tell me that's enough and it was time to go back. I would protest in my defense that I couldn't stop, and the pain was agonizing. Followed by making more multiple fart noises. When I came out of the bathroom, I would usually have the biggest smirk on my face and sometimes crack up laughing at myself. She would always look at me laughing and would say "Jason McLean, you are something else." She was not wrong.

The first psychologist that was sent in to analyze me might as well have been a textbook with arms and legs. Possessing the wonderful personality qualities of a dead fish and a face that I wanted to punch. This man would talk to me, not with me. That was apparent upfront. It felt as though when he asked me questions, he didn't even listen to my answers. It was like a robot that had been preprogrammed ahead of time, very automated in his approach. Near the end of our first meeting, I pretended to fall asleep and made snoring noises hoping he would wrap it up. He gave me a textbook description of my behavior which was so exhilarating and profound. We called it a day. As he left my cavern he said, "today went well." "I said I already feel cured of all that's wrong with me. It's a miracle," closing my eyes once again and pretending to fall asleep. Later that night I found a couple books on psychology, sociology, and philosophy that my dad still had from a previous attempt at university. I read and memorized them as best I could. Making a few notes for myself along the way. Fascinating stuff.

The next meeting with Johnny Textbook and associates was our last. I would reply to all his questions with linguistic relativity, meaning basically I would say things to influence his perception and thoughts which would affect his behavior or approach, essentially causing him to derail from the tracks of his train of thought. Brilliantly mischievous on my part. This would continue throughout the next few walking textbooks I was forced to meet with and talk to.

Child and Family Services got involved as well. One Monday morning I was told that a social worker was coming that day to meet with me. I immediately began to plan my strategy to make this person want to quit on me, as the others before had. About an hour later, enter John Smith. A tall man with dark feathered hair, glasses, casually dressed and a very distinguished moustache, I mean that thing was thick. It was like a chinchilla on his top lip. His voice was soft, and he spoke in a way to me that was prodigiously different from the others before him. It actually seemed as though John Smith listened to what we talked about and did not immediately dissect everything I said into regurgitated psychiatric terminology. He seemed patient, interested, genuine and most importantly, without judgement. He asked me mainly about what I liked and what I was good at. My hobbies. Nothing to do with my family, my issues, my struggles at all. I told him that I loved drawing. I loved animals and studying them. I liked solving mazes. Reading Marvel comic books. Playing hockey. And of course, Ninjitsu. I was actively training to become a ninja in my bedroom and backyard. With the hopes of taking that to the next level of perhaps somehow becoming a jedi as well. He asked me what it was that I liked so much about those things, and he undoubtedly cared about hearing my answers.

As things wrapped up in our introductory meeting, John asked me if it was ok with me that we met again to talk. I optimistically agreed with that. For the first time, I admittedly looked forward to our ensuing meeting.

As our meetings went on for the next few weeks John would read X Men comic books with me and ask me to explain to him what I thought was going on in them and if I related to them. He would bring mazes and watch me do them and then eventually started timing me to see how fast I could solve them. He liked to play games with me that tested my intellect and problem solving. For each new meeting he would ask me to draw him an animal as lifelike as possible and write a very descriptive breakdown of that animal's particular characteristics. John then asked for permission from the school, psychologist, and my parents if he could take me out for a couple hours every week. I had been increasing my level of commitment to my schoolwork and since John had shown up, I had not had any outbursts or been disruptive either. I had become more focused on controlling myself because if I had a meltdown, I knew I would not get to see John that week. John was granted three hours a week to take me somewhere and he had to provide an analysis of my behavior after every outing. I had been a good little animal. Let the celebrations begin!

The first place we went was the Zoo. It was only about a fifteen-minute drive from my school, so we got to spend the greater majority of the allotted time there. I remember being so excited when we got there. Feeling so grateful for John Smith's dedication to me. We would walk through the zoo, and I would tell him all about the animals, what they ate, where they lived in the wild, if they were a predator or prey, if they worked in a pack or were a solo animal. As we continued walking John every once and awhile would ask me a question that was related to the other animals related to how I felt about certain things like school, my teachers, my friends, and my family. He was subtle and slick, and he got his answers. Never once did he interrupted me, did not tell me I was wrong, didn't use fancy words and most of all, he never had to be right in his explanations. He always asked me if it was okay to share his thoughts which were never confrontational or pressuring. I often shared with him how I related to the wild animals trapped in their cages. How they paced just like I did, back and forth, always looking for a way to escape to where they belonged. To run wild. To be free again.

We would return to the zoo many more times. Each time was better than the last. Once, he took me for ice cream which I really enjoyed. He was very creatively clever in his game plan, constantly empowering me to want to talk to him about many of the issues I was struggling with. He took me to the Faculty of Science, the Department of Biology and Zoology at the University of Manitoba. I had the privilege of meeting Professors of the department and had the opportunity to share my knowledge and passion about Zoology with them. I was shown all kinds of incredible samples of preserved species, some observations into scientific experiments that were being done there for enhanced agriculture, live ecosystems and I even got to interact with a two headed snake. I was in biology heaven. I noticed that one of the professors and John had been talking quite a bit and John was writing down some notes in his pocketbook notepad. When we were driving back to my school, I asked him what the notes he was taking down were about. He looked at me with a smile and told me that the Professor I met was very impressed with me and stated to John that I was incredibly full of knowledge. That he found it difficult to believe that I was having so many challenges at school with the higher level of intellect I had shown. John was proud of me and that felt good.

After submitting his report on that outing, John had recommended to the school staff and my parents to have the child psychologist administer an Aptitude Test to better understand my capability for learning in order to set up some strategic plans to help further my education.

Our next meeting, the psychologist and John explained the fundamentals of the test. He asked me to apply myself and answer the questions as best that I could, and not to worry about how many questions I answered correctly or incorrectly. He explained to me that this test would help to clarify where my strengths and weaknesses were cognitively. To provide insight into any challenges that might hinder my learning capacity. John then looked at me with a big smile and a sparkle in his eye and said "Jason, I want you to prove to yourself how smart you really are so nobody can tell you otherwise ever again."

Bing! The biggest and brightest light bulb lit up in my brain and when I looked at that test, I saw everything in a new light. I was not afraid to fail. I completed the very intellectually imposing test. John looked at me and asked me how I thought I did? I answered with a smirk on my face "pretty good."

Later that week the Psychologist shared my results with John, The School Staff, and my parents. Stating that I somehow cheated because in many categories I had scored higher than the average university student, even higher in the visual problem solving and sciences categories. My knowledge of mathematics and mathematical problem solving were lower than the average for a ten-year-old. When my dad told me about the test results, they asked me if I had cheated. I remember being so heartbroken when he asked me that. I asked him why they thought I cheated? My dad explained to me that I scored very high on the test, and they didn't believe I was able to do so. I asked my dad if he thought I cheated and then I asked if John thought the same. My dad looked at me and said that John had called him stating that there was no way I cheated and that my dad believed him. My dad attempted to rationalize the reasoning behind the accusation. He told me that they wanted me to take a re-test and asked me if I would be willing to do so. The answer was a redemptional YES.

When I sat down in my cage to take the re-test, the psychologist, guidance counselor and John Smith all stayed in the room with me. To ensure that I did not cheat on this test. The usual distractions that shattered my concentration were all present but became nonexistent to me at that moment. As the talking textbook was babbling about whatever, his voice made me sick to my stomach, angry and vengeful. I rudely interrupted him and said, "just give me the test and do not talk to me again." I stared at him with a fierce gaze, I wanted to rip his face off, my eyes colder than ice as he passed me the new set of test papers to me. I would not even acknowledge my Guidance Counselor, not looking at her once. The moment before I started to write the test, I looked at John Smith and said, "thank you for believing in me, when no one else did." From that point on, I focused all my anger and pain into every single question. Totally dialing into every detail of all the hundreds of questions, memory tests, geometrical problem solving, verbal and visual comprehension problem solving, analogies, classification, mathematics, general knowledge, and logic. The mathematical questions seemed to be more difficult this time round. I remember feeling that the questions on this test were different and unquestionably more challenging than the last, but I would not let that phase me. After completion, I sat there staring straight ahead at the wall across from me, not saying a word until they were leaving. John asked me if we were still on for our regular scheduled meeting the next day and I nodded. I then said to the three that" the test they had given me was not the same test as before. Totally different questions and subjects. Nice try though."

Class dismissed.

The next meeting would include my parents, all the usual characters from the school. This meeting was to go over the results of the Re-test and discuss it. John Smith seemed quite ecstatic upon his entrance. As John began speaking it was very evident that he had good news. He stated that I scored even higher than the previous test including in some areas of mathematics. John also declared that the physiologist had mistakenly handed me a test suitable for university level students, not the children's version that I had finalized before. He asked me how I scored so outstanding on a test that was so much more complex and challenging. My answer was simple. I was extremely mad that everybody thought I cheated on the first test. I wanted to show my dad and John that they were right in believing in me. My anger became the instrument which funneled my determination and focus. I took the time at every question or problem and broke it down into the smallest of components. I reworked it and rebuilt it until I understood the question congruously. I also recognized patterns in the questions and used that to my advantage. Which made the answer come to life like sheet lightning flashing from cloud to cloud in the sky of my mind. John Smith explained to the group that I had surpassed university levels on this test with the exception of mathematics, although showed increased improvement in mathematical problem solving. Everyone found out that day that the dumb loud problem child was a smarty pants. Break out the Bunsen burners and beakers.

Let the experiments on the guinea pig begin

CHAPTER 6

WHERE THE STREETS HAVE NO NAME

An empty stomach, an empty wallet and a broken heart can teach you the best lessons of life.
Robin Williams

I remember overhearing the conversation that the "renowned" child psychiatrist/ psychotherapist shared with my parents after I had been meeting with him on the regular. The conversation had dire expectations of any success for me in my future life. The man who was informing my parents of the doomsday scenario of my future was an arrogant narcissist who never listened to anything I said and at no time came across as compassionate. I found him to be rude and pompous as he spoke in a very condescending way anytime, I asked him questions. I felt belittled by him and his know-it-all approach to our conversations. He would explain that I would never be able to finish school, I would not ever be capable of maintaining a healthy relationship, lifestyle, or job. I would need to live with my parents for the rest of my life because I would be a failure otherwise, unable to take care of myself. I would most likely end up on the streets or in jail, I would never amount to anything due to his diagnosis of my mental illnesses. I was reduced to a collection of acronyms for mental illness that then defined me. His advice for my parents was to kick me out of the house and not let me back in anytime I continued to behave erratically and was not able to control my emotions, and to call the police if I refused to leave or if I got violent. If I ran away not to let me in. No matter what the circumstances were. To call the police on me if I persisted in attempting to come home. Both my mother and father were remarried, and this was to stand on both sides of the family as the treatment to help me get better. He spoke to my parents like I was not in the room, like I was not there. I perceived this like I was not to understand what was being said or that what I thought or felt was meaningless and of no significance. It was at that moment that my life was reduced to nothing, and I died inside. I was fourteen years old.

Looking back at my life, I have always contemplated the idea that if I my future had not been so negatively forecasted by that psychotherapist, would my life have taken a different direction and not followed in suit of his projected prognosis. In retrospect, impressionable young me gave up on future me, that day. I became a tornado of anger, pain and depression that wildly spun uncontrollably, and all hell broke loose.

76 CARS

When I was a teenager, I spent a lot of time on the streets. I would run away from home constantly and then when I did come home, I was so out of control that no one could handle me anymore. My parents did what they could to try and help me, but by that point I was doing so many drugs and drinking that my mind was severely jeopardized. My symptoms from my mental illnesses were catching and spreading through me like a wildfire. I was uncontrollable and violent, like a cannonball smashing through a hundred walls made of glass.

Being homeless as a teenage boy was terrifying and challenged everything, I thought about every second. I was not prepared for being homeless, but I had no other choice than to make a permanent shift into survival mode. I spent many days and nights alone walking the streets downtown, in parks, looking for somewhere safe to rest. Winnipeg is a very violent and unforgiving city. Cell phones did not exist back then. I had no way to contact anyone unless I rigged a payphone. Making it impossible to communicate with anyone late at night to find somewhere to stay. There was no navigation to help you find somewhere to go. I often was followed, chased, attacked, and beat up. Some nights it was the cops, laying a beating on me and then driving away, leaving me there crumpled over in pain. Other nights it was a group of drunk men cutting through somewhere after the bar and then they spotted me. The chase was on. I ran as fast as I could but sometimes, they caught up to me, taking turns laying the boots to me. Hard to fight back when you have not eaten. Hard to run with no fuel in the tank. I was followed by men late at night that looked like their intentions were that of sexual violence against me. Sometimes ending in a physical confrontation, where I would smash my fists into their heads until the muscles in my arms could no longer allow me to do so. Making sure they would think twice before following me or anyone else again. Other times I avoided conflict by running away. I had knives pulled on me often, even a gun on a couple occasions. There were violent street gangs downtown and avoiding them because I was all alone most of the time was a nightly endeavor. Some nights I would sleep at a friend's place. Those were the best nights. I felt safe, I was warm, I went to sleep all night and didn't worry until the next day started. I basically lived in one of my best lifelong friends' basements for about three months before his family even knew I was there. It was a very large house on Lamont Street in the fancy pants area of Tuxedo. There were always great leftovers in the fridge which was a big bonus. His family were very kind and generous once they got to know me, making me feel as though I was a welcome addition to their already large family. A few years later in that same basement, one of his older brothers would take his life in a heartbreaking tragedy that ripped our lives in half. He had been battling mental illness and fought as hard as he could.

The nights when I couldn't find a place to stay, those were the scary ones. They lasted forever. I slept in heated underground lots, I broke into cars to escape the rain or snow, I would hide in heated parking lots between cars, I was sleeping in half-built houses that were under construction, I would build a makeshift shelter out of plywood and off cuts and of lumber and use bundles of insulation to keep out of the wind, rain, or snow. When it was warmer, outdoor hockey rinks were usually safe places to rest at night, tucking myself in the penalty box which offered out of sight close quarters and a break from the wind. I remember sleeping in the Pan Am Pool building for almost three weeks. A massive building constructed for the Pan American games many years previous. I slept under a set of concrete stairs on the second floor close to the track that looped around the pool. I would be out of sight there if I crammed in under the canopy of concrete. I would sneak into the pool just before close and hide until the staff left. Lucky for me, I suppose way back when technology and security was in a stage of infancy. There weren't motion detectors or cameras. After a few nights of sleeping under the same stairs one night when I returned and was going to my hiding spot there were a couple of chocolate bars and bags of chips waiting for me under the stairs. I ate them so fast; I was so hungry, I was starving. I hadn't eaten that day at all. The night cleaner had seen me, he never disturbed me, he never asked me to leave. Instead, every night I would find snacks and comic books there. He never woke me up, never tried to talk to me. I guess he just understood and did his part to help me out.

One time my sister snuck me into my mom's house where I wasn’t allowed to be anymore due to my wild behavior. I had stolen things from their house and had become hostile towards my mom and her husband. That night I slept in the basement on the cold concrete floor on top of a towel in my winter clothing. I would take that over walking the streets any night.

Winnipeg had an extremely long cold snap at that time. Being in a humid continental climate zone, the winter and summer can be very extreme in its seasonal conditions. It was a true minus thirty degrees Celsius for many consecutive nights or colder. Back then when the temperature was stated, it was the actual temperature before the windchill. With the windchill warning it was somewhere between minus forty to minus fifty degrees. Colder than the Arctic. In fact, as cold as the surface on the planet Mars. One night that I will never forget, it had dropped to minus thirty-seven and with the windchill, it was minus fifty. A ferociously gusting north wind that punched me relentlessly in the face as a boxer would constantly remind me of the bitterness of temperature. I had been walking for about two hours trying to stay alive. To keep moving. I knew that there wasn't a chance of me dying if I stopped moving and froze, it was irrefutable that I would freeze to death if I did. I was trying to get to the Salisbury House restaurant in Tuxedo, where it was open twenty-four hours and a tough looking, smart talking woman named Sheila worked there and would often let me sit inside and stay warm all night. Sheila would always treat me to a coffee and a piece of wafer pie which was the best. She had a goofy laugh and although a tough exterior, she had a huge heart of gold. I was less than a half a kilometer away when I began to feel my brain start to shut down, my feet were like solid rocks without any feeling. My eyes were freezing shut. I was beyond exhausted and dehydrated. My voice slurred and sounded like I was talking in slow motion, as I was trying to talk out loud to myself to stay alert. To stay awake. To stay alive. That ended quicker than a tick in a New York minute. I became drowsy and clumsy, like I was very intoxicated. I was losing all coordination. I lied down on a bus bench in hopes of resting my tired body. The wooden back support of the bench acted like a wind break. I kept telling myself to not fall asleep, because if I did, I knew I would not wake up. I remember vividly feeling so alone. Invisible. Lost. Unwanted.

I started counting cars out loud to stay awake, to keep my brain as active as possible. What was amazing for me in this moment when I look back at it was that I could actually keep focus on the number of cars I counted. I have ADHD and normally I am unable to count to ten in my head without losing track and have to start the counting process over. This made it very tough for me to count sheep at night in hopes of falling asleep, instead presenting a very discouraging experience. Perhaps it was due to certain parts of my brain malfunctioning due to the onslaught of hypothermia and somehow another area of the brain was able to perform this function out of survival mode. I counted seventy-six cars that drove by me, that included cars travelling in both directions. Not one single person stopped to ask if I needed help, if there was somewhere they could take me, and invited me to come warm up inside their vehicle if I was ok. not one person got out of their car to check if I was still alive. Every single one of them were fully aware of the extreme dangerous temperatures and that on the news that evening they had been warning people to stay inside. I'm positive that some didn't notice me as they drove by. At least that's what I told myself. To this day I often wonder if there was a cute dog on that same bench, that same night in that same deadly cold weather, freezing to death. How many cars out of the seventy-six that I counted before losing consciousness would have pulled over and at least let the dog in their warm vehicle and try to figure out a way to get it to safety while the young dog was warming up. I wondered how many would have said to themselves or the other people in their car that the poor dog is going to freeze to death, we have to help it, or it will die. I'm all for rescuing dogs, I have rescued a few myself and adopted some as well. I think that it is a truly wonderful thing and have encouraged every person I know that wants to get a dog to adopt a rescue. I would be curious to know that if people treated people like dogs in need of rescuing, would that change the world we live in? Would a new enlightened level of open-minded compassion dramatically influence people's train of thought when seeing someone on the streets? Perhaps opening their eyes to see that is a person just like them or like someone they love. Someone's mother, grandfather, husband, sister, brother, friend, instead of someone who is wasted, junked out, disgusting, dirty, crazy, or pathetic as commonly mis conceptualized. Imagine if everyone opened their mind and realized that at one time those people living on the streets actually didn't before. The streets were the only available landing pad when they had been torn away from the life they once had. Whether it had been from tragedy, mental illness, trauma, broken homes, abuse, addictions, lack of affordable housing, unemployment, escaping violent or abusive relationships, skyrocketing costs of living or devastating economic situations causing extreme poverty invoking a vicious cycle that is almost impossible to climb out of financially once in it. Constantly being exposed to the indecency of the uncertain life that is theirs. Or is it simply more convenient to continue driving and pretend we don't see anyone so we can sleep better at night in our warm bed?

The seventy-seventh car I called it, and it may have been more than that as I was in and out of consciousness and possibly seeing double, was a taxicab driven by a man. He got out of his cab and walked over to me asking some questions about why I was out in the freezing cold all by myself, but I was succumbing to hypothermia and unable to speak properly. I do remember he had kind sincere eyes with a terribly concerned look upon his face. I can also vaguely remember thinking to myself that I had no money for a cab ride as I drifted off into the freezing cold darkness losing consciousness again. I was woken up abruptly by him pushing hard down on my chest. He was performing CPR on me as he thought I had stopped breathing. The dangerous crisis that severe hypothermia presents is that the body temperature lowers to a life-threatening level while the body can no longer produce enough heat to maintain a safe operating temperature which slows down breathing and can lead to brain malfunction, cardiac arrest, and death. The cab driver had taken me to a hospital that was nearby, about a ten-minute drive. I do not remember the ride there. I remember my clothes being taken off me by panicked nurses, being wrapped in warm blankets and hot pockets, a heating lamp, and IV running a warm saline solution in an attempt to heat up my blood. I overheard mumblings from a doctor stating that they may have to amputate some of my fingers and possibly my feet. I can still remember to this day the excruciating pain of my tissue thawing out and my nerve endings sending electrifying feelings like I was on fire, making the idea of freezing to death not such a bad option after all. Oddly amid all the disarray, I felt safe and comfortable as I was being attended to by the staff at the hospital. They put my health and safety first but soon enough the questions all began to arise from the nurses about who I was and why I was all alone out in the cold. I lied to them and provided a fake name and age; I had no identification on me to prove otherwise telling the staff that I had lost my wallet. Stating that I had just moved from a different province and was staying with a friend. I knew from experience that if they found out I was under eighteen that Child and Family Services would be called in and I did not want that to happen. Although they may have had my best interests at heart, the idea of another placement or foster home made me sick to my stomach. I would have rather puked up metal coat hangers than go through that. I just wanted to be with my family even though that seemed to be an impossible dream. Over the course of the next two days my skin changed color to a very darkened blueish purple on my feet and hands blowing up with massive painful blisters from severe frostbite. Amputation was ruled out which brought a feeling of immense relief from what could have been a gruesome repercussion from an already harrowing experience. Consequently, I had thought to myself that maybe this traumatic experience was the one to trigger my mutation and release the ability of super healing as my body had shown miraculous recovery bringing me one step closer to becoming Wolverine, my hero from the X-Men.

PEANUT BUTTER PACKETS

There was this popular greasy spoon, mom, and pop restaurant downtown. Inside, it looked like a small cafeteria, not much for decor and wreaked of garlic and oils used in cooking very delicious breakfasts. A welcoming scent for a hungry stomach. Every morning I would casually walk through the restaurant saying hello to people and I would steal handfuls of peanut butter packets and different types of jams, filling my pockets with as many of them as I could. The packets that were on the tables were usually in a stainless-steel holder or on a small plate and there to put on your toast with your breakfast. I would take these because the peanut butter ones were very high in protein, rich with fat and calories. I love peanut butter. It's hard to eat peanut butter fast. When you're starving because you have not eaten in a day and you have only slept for two or three hours, you become so hungry that your stomach feels like it's literally crawling out of your esophagus trying to get food conjointly you feel so empty inside from hunger that you can barely walk or think. I would try to eat those peanut butter packets as fast as I could. If you have a dog or have seen someone feed a dog peanut butter, you know that it takes a little while to take it down. The same goes for a human being, but it would give me enough protein and fat that I could have some energy and my mind was able to slowly reset and commence thinking clearer. The jam had lots of sugars, carbohydrates, and some vitamins. Making it a wonderful dessert after feasting on peanut butter. It was not much, but it served its purpose as life support. I was always quite skinny and small growing up, but at this point I looked like a walking skeleton, just skin and bones.

One morning I walked slowly into that same restaurant, surveying the entire room. It was just after the early morning breakfast rush when I arrived. The lady that cooked on the grill looked up at me and immediately she said come here. Gesturing with her hand to come closer. I paused and didn't move towards her because I thought she was going to yell at me or call the police like a lot of other places had, as I made the rounds of many restaurants downtown daily. She looked at me with caring eyes and asked "are you hungry? I see you come in here and take those peanut butters. That can't be enough to fill up your stomach." I looked at her like a deer caught in the headlights of a car in the dark of night on a remote highway. She asked me what I wanted for breakfast and that she would take care of it. No charge. It was on the house. I remember smiling so big that it felt like it was going to crack my cold face. So naturally I ordered the biggest breakfast special they had. I ordered a glass of chocolate milk to wash it down, the hungry man's breakfast with extra bacon and a side of pancakes. She looked at me with a big kind smile that was warm and nurturing and asked me when the last time I ate was. I just looked at her and I can still recall feeling all the tears building up in my eyes. I sat down at a table facing away from the rest of the people in the restaurant because I did not want anyone to see me cry. After a few minutes, she sat down with me when she brought over my food, and she told me that I didn't have to come and steal things anymore. She told me that she would make me breakfast anytime if I was willing to clean up tables and wash dishes afterwards for an hour or two. I happily agreed to that on the spot. Motivated by all the stacks of pancakes I could eat. The sweet lady asked me where I lived, and I just shook my head. Her eyes were saddened, "where are your parents? Do you have family here?" she asked. I replied "I do, but I am too out of control and bad. All I do is hurt everybody. I can't control my anger. I steal from them, and I don't know why I do it. I run away and then try to go back but the same thing always happens. I can't do anything right and nobody knows what's wrong with me." She looked at me sadly for a second and then smiled at me. She said, "I'm sure your parents love you very much but sometimes people have to show tough love to get through to the people they love the most and maybe that's what they're doing now." I can only imagine how hard it was for my parents to go through this as well.

Later, after I finished washing dishes and helping clean up the place, I remember thinking how kind of a woman that she was, and I imagined she had a son as well. Perchance, I reminded her of him. I left there feeling renewed. I felt noticed. I was excited to go back the next day. I had a full stomach too! I also thought about stealing more peanut butter packets but stopped myself, perhaps my default way of survival thinking was kicking in.

The extraordinarily paradoxical thing about all of this experience was that I actually went into that restaurant that morning to rob it at knifepoint. I knew they had a lot of cash in the till every morning from all the people that ate breakfast there as it was quite a popular spot. Everyone paid in cash back then. I had a large military survival hunting knife on me with a nine-inch blade that one side was serrated like shark teeth. Just as I was about to start to reach for the knife was the exact same second that she started her conversation with me, offering me breakfast. That is why I was so stunned when it happened. I always wondered if she knew what I was up to. She must have recognized something wasn't right with me. Perhaps she saw the eyes of a young boy about to do something really bad that could have had lifelong repercussions. Life altering consequences. It's amazing how things happen like that in life. What could have happened that day if I had robbed the place at knifepoint if I ended up stabbing someone out of panic or ran from the police and potentially got shot down in my haste to escape the scene of the crime. It's safe to say that a random act of kindness with perfect timing can completely change even the most evil and diabolical plan. I now believe that any act of kindness is done so in the immaculate timeframe of exactly when it should take place. In this case, maybe it was because she saw the two policemen walking in the door behind me to order their breakfast in which I had no idea they had entered the restaurant and were standing there. Either way, retrospectively, I look back upon the experience as a miracle. A life defining moment that taught me one of the most valuable lessons. No matter how bad things are in life, unconditional kindness can literally change everything in a single heartbeat. The blink of an eye. Every act of kindness holds the power to make any moment become radiant, outshining the darkness that the previous moment eclipsed.

BIRDS OF A FEATHER

The world is a horrifyingly ruthless place when you're all alone and have nowhere to go, nowhere to eat, nowhere to sleep and it seems as though nobody cares about you anymore. You have no name. The streets all blend into one, as do the days and nights. Desperation quickly becomes the dictator of how time is spent. That time can slow down as though it seems that the hardest loneliest moments will never ever end. Expanding the pain and suffering that you feel to a point that it is debilitating. Losing yourself inside your looping state of lost hope. The same can be said for mental illness. There is no doubt that living on the streets instituted deep rooted psychological damages and caused mayhem in my mind for many years afterwards. Revealing a true reflection in the mirror of society regarding mental illness and those being homeless. Unfortunately, the greater majority of judgements focus on those poor souls that are perceived to have crossed over into the point of no return with drugs and alcohol, schizophrenia or hit rock bottom. Imagine taking a long cold lonely walk in their shoes, that their souls are full of holes and have worn so thin.

I can tell you from experience it's a place that you have never wanted to have been. I was trapped there and would return there a few more times in my twenties. Bouncing from place to place. Group of friends to new group of friends. Job to job. I lived in a van for many long months. Stealing trendy clothing regularly so I could look like I had money by the way I dressed when I was out and about. Working all day and then showering at the YMCA afterwards until I got myself back on track. In my early twenties I would start sending violent messages to people for money, collecting unpaid debts and as well supplying drugs to those in need. Only to become more tightly entangled in a web of alcohol and drug abuse, anger, violence, and self-destruction.

It was there that I found myself a new family in the welcoming arms of street gangs. Brothers of a new kind. A place where I thought it felt like I belonged. I felt accepted. Where my violence was celebrated, and my crazy ways were standard issue. I was part of a pack. Weaponizing my anger and enhancing the focal point of my rage more rapidly every day. I wanted to make people afraid of me. I wanted revenge on all those who scarred me, altered me, and stole pieces of me away and discarded them just like they were throwing out the garbage. Pieces I thought I could only get back by inflicting pain upon them.

My toxic relationship with steroids began here. I had tried steroids a couple times previously but in my mid-twenties into my thirties I packed on close to fifty pounds of lean muscle mass while becoming addicted to steroids and other related drugs. Becoming more menacing and vicious with the increases of testosterone and multiple other steroids that I stacked with. Building the colossal armor around the scared little boy, I decorated my armor with tattoos. Colorful warnings like those dangerous animals wear in the wild to let others know their deadly nature. To stay away or feel the wrath of my anger. Many people got hurt because they ignored my warnings. My insecurities from being bullied as a kid were always there in every fight I fought, and I fought a lot. I was in well over a hundred street fights, bar fights, and gang fights. That number is not even inclusive of all the people I beat up that owed money, slept with the wrong girl, or had done something they should not have done to someone I cared about. A little fearful child's voice in my head would tell me to run away instead of fighting someone every time. Then a switch would flick and the voice of that frightened child in my head turned to animosity in the voice of the boy who wanted revenge on all those who had hurt him in the past. In a split second I flipped from scared to psychotic and the wild beast was unleashed.

I was living two very different lives. One life was a life that was fairly normal on paper I suppose. I had a job. I had a girlfriend. I had friends. I liked to have a good time. I was in the gym often lifting weights and practiced different martial arts. Visited with my family. A normal life it would seem to the untrained eye.

The other life I was living was quite the antithetical. Gang life. Money, power, violence, partying, sex, drugs, alcohol, and all the dangerously encompassing environments that wildlife presented. It was such a subversive rush of fury and lust. My life could have ended at any time as I was always at risk of retaliation from rivals. I was abusing cocaine, prescription painkillers, and alcohol routinely. The potential for danger and harm were always present no matter how precocious I thought I was. I was always out all the time, in bars, parties, restaurants. We were revered and feared. People flocked to us everywhere we went. I quickly became addicted to all these things, and even more so the feelings that took me away from who I was struggling inside to be. My ego developed into a new identity overnight it seemed. A split personality that seemingly managed my two very distinctly antagonistic lifestyles accordingly in conjunction with each other. In reality it was a masterful delusion orchestrated behind the scenes in a theatrical production put on by my mental illness. I was in a state of constant conflict and crisis. I would rip myself apart when I was alone. I could not handle the emotional repercussions of my wildlife and its violent conduct. I inadvertently attempted to desensitize with substance abuse. Alcohol and drugs became a domineering habit with me as I used them as a way to escape from the conflict within myself, it only got worse as I became more addicted to the high, I obtained from the rush of my lifestyle whilst mutually benumbing the feelings of guilt, anger, and bitterness that I thought I was escaping from when high and drunk. As time went on, the highs diminished quickly as the lows dramatically increased in volume and destructive force. The bridge that separated my two lifestyles caught on fire and was incinerated as I was unable to contain the spreading of hellfire within my head. I was becoming more violent, reckless, and depressed. The endless nights, the fears, the anxiety were all compiling. I was spinning webs of self-deceit that I was getting caught up in, self-destructive traps that I wove for myself. The pressures that were upon me from all directions of my life exposed a very small crack in my armor. Where there was an opportunity for a sliver of guiding light to shine inside my armor through that tiny crack and illuminate a way out of it, like a lighthouse in the fog of a stormy sea. I wanted to wrap the light around me and expand it as big as my life. Instead, all I saw was ink black darkness that surrounded the light and then consumed it. Smashing that window of opportunity. There was no escape for me. I had become my own most dangerous enemy.

CHAPTER 7

THE DARK SIDE OF THE MOUNTAIN

Fear is the path to the dark side. Fear leads to anger, anger leads to hate, hate leads to suffering.
Yoda, Jedi Master

There the old man stood. Finally stopped running. He had been running away for as long as he could remember. Running in the same direction for all his life but never getting anywhere new. It was not his idea to stop there, but an obstacle forced him to do so. There in his path stood a giant. Staring down directly at him. In fact, it was so big and monstrous it blocked out sunlight, casting a massive shadow across its colossal north facing foothold. Its outstretched encumbrance was as far as one could see, from the east to the west. This gargantuan monstrosity was composed of sharp ridges, jagged ledges, treacherous cliffs, near vertical slopes of dark granite and mountain sides made of protruding and impaling rocks shaped like massive spears.

As he stood there in awe analyzing the massive obstacle before him. In its ominous appearance there was no way around the mountain. Looking from the base upwards to its summit, it would be impossible to climb all the way to the top. It would be a suicidal mission he thought to himself.

So, the old man sat down in front of the silent giant. Feeling sorry for himself he started saying things under his breath like "why does this always happen to me?", "I can never win", "nothing ever goes my way." He looked up and cursed at the sky above. As he sat there longer and longer, he grew more and more upset with his situation. There was no way to get around the mountain and the climb would surely kill him. He had convinced himself of this. The old man kept looking all the way to the highest peaks and telling himself there is no way he could do it. What if he was only able to climb partway up and then become too weak to continue, starving to death in agony, all alone. The rocks are like knives, what if he got badly cut and bleed to death. No one will ever find him except for the vultures and whatever carnivorous creatures lurk in the dark caves and shadows. He thought to himself what if he got ate to death? What if there are deadly scorpions, massive spiders, vicious snakes, vampire bats flying out of the caves at night. What if he lost his footing and fell to my doom? He thought of every possible scenario in which he failed to survive the climb and his thoughts began to spin uncontrollably. He broke down and started crying. He could see absolutely nothing past the moment in which he was imprisoned. Wallowing in his misery only added to his self-defeating demise at the base of the dark side of the mountain. Then his anger set in. He knew freedom was on the other side of the mountain. But he could not obtain it. There was just no possible way. He would perish with only his thoughts as he had nothing to eat, no water to drink and was growing weaker by the minutes that passed him by. The risk involved far outweighed the reward in his mind he had sadly convinced himself. Even though there was no way to go back, he remained immobilized, Frozen in fear. Paralysis in panic. The more he thought about climbing the mountainous obstruction, the more he fed into all the fears of the things that could go wrong. Fueling his fear so rapidly, it spread like wildfire. Doubt, due to not believing in himself, had cemented his fate. Sealing the last nail in his coffin. So, he sat there mentally disabling himself and in fear and anger he began to hate his life, hate the world and the people in it, especially the ones who were happy and living their lives in a manner in which they desired. He hated the heavens above for never setting him free. He blamed everything and everyone for his failures, his losses, his life never becoming what he wanted it to be. He gave up and suffered the consequences.

A day had passed, and the old man sat there slowly dying in his misery. He had dislocated himself from all hope and became complacent dying there. Later in the afternoon that day, he was lying on his back staring up at the great mountain that loomed over him. When suddenly, out of nowhere, a young boy was walking towards him. The old man sat up trying to focus his eyes on the young boy. He asked himself was this a delusion, was his imagination playing tricks on him? The boy approached the old man and greeted him with energy and enthusiasm like that of someone who had all the life within him. The young boy asked "are you hungry? Are you thirsty? I have some fruit and I have water." The boy was wearing a small pouch which contained some fruit, a couple canteens full of water. The old man was in disbelief but was also starving and dying of thirst. He grabbed and ate the apple; he grabbed the boy's canteen and began to drink the water. The young boy interrupted him saying we must save that because we have a long way to go. We can't drink at all right now. The boy looked into the man's green eyes and then turned and faced the Dark Side of the Mountain. The young boy looked up the mountain surveying all its peaks and ridges. He could see in his mind all the way to the very top up the mountain. He then looked at the old man and with a big smile. The boy excitedly said, "get up, we have a mountain to climb!" The old man shouted at the boy "there is no way to climb to the top! It's impossible!" "Go home, before you hurt yourself!" barked the old man to the boy. The boy retorted "I have no home to go to, it's been long gone. I think there will be a home for me that will be revealed once we climb to the very top and can see what's on the other side of this mountain. A new beginning!"

The old man sat there miserable staring at the boy. He was exhausted, beaten up and down for the count. The old man had no fight left in him. He was too scared to stand up and give it one last shot. The boy's energy was contagious. The young boy said to the old man "I'm going to climb this mountain with or without you. If we work as a team, there's no doubt in my mind that we can get to the top of this mountain together. Just imagine how amazing of an accomplishment that will be and how powerful we will feel when we stand on the very summit of this gargantuan mountain. We can look back to where we started and look at all the different moments in which we worked to get to the very top and are now facing the most beautiful unknown in front of us." The boy then stated that he had enough water to last us for a couple days. I have a variety of fruits that will provide us with energy and keep our stomachs full."

The old man let out a deep sigh, looking into the green eyes of the young boy that looked just like his. "I'm afraid I'll die climbing this mountain. So, there is no point for me to even try." The boy's face lit up with an encouraging smile and he said "It looks to me that you've already died right here, so what do you have to lose in climbing this mountain? At least then you'll die from attempting to accomplish a great quest."

The boy reached out his hand and asked the old man "will you please join me, together we can do this, I promise you." A tear slowly rolled down the old man's face. He sighed and said" fine, at least I'll have your company, that's better than dying alone I suppose. We will have to go slowly up the mountain" proclaimed the old man. The young boy smiled and replied "Slow and steady we go my captain"

As they reached the highest peak of the mountain after a couple days of climbing, the old man's energy and vigor were restored to what it once was many years before. He had become grateful through this journey up this unclimbable mountain that led to the unknown. The old man sat down. He began to cry out tears of joy, tears of anguish. Tears he had held back his entire life. Teardrops that fell heavily and happily. The young boy joined him by his side. They both marveled in their triumph as they looked down the treacherous mountain they had climbed together. They looked at the fascinating view in front of them, rich and abundant with light and life, as far as they could see. They were literally feeling on top of the world as the old man looked to the boy and said "you are an amazing mountain climber! How many mountains have you climbed to be so skilled and undaunted?" The boy cracked up in laughter. He said "thank you! I'll be honest with you; this is the very first mountain I have ever climbed!" The old man's eyes opened wide, and a look of disbelief was painted on his face. "What?!" questioned the old man. If you have never climbed a mountain before, how were you not scared to climb this beast?" How were you able to calibrate a plan to overcome such odds of survival?" The boy gazed out towards the sunshine in the horizon with a grin. "I had no other mountain to compare it to in my mind. I had not experienced climbing a mountain before. I was never taught the dangers of mountain climbing by anyone. So, when I looked at the mountain, I only saw an opportunity to climb the mountain. That climbing this mountain would take me somewhere I have not been. To the unknown which I would cradle. I believed that I could do it. It is really that elementary. Instead of thinking about all that could go wrong and talking myself out of it, I simply thought about all that would go right, if I believed in myself. At that point the mountain was no longer the obstacle in which to conquer. The obstacle remaining to be vanquished was fear. Not fear of the mountain itself, but fear of the unknown, fear of failure, fear of succeeding when we do not believe we deserve it, fear of separation and finally the fear of death. Once you overcome that, you will possess the perspective that you found something that you would die for, which in turn gives the true meaning in what you live for. Once all manufactured fear of failure is relinquished, you will truly live a free life."

The old man was astonished by the young boy's wisdom and wanted to know how a child could know so much. "Earlier you had said to me that you have no home, that it was long gone. How could that be? Where is your family? I never even asked you, ``What is your name, boy?" asked the old man. The boy smiled at the old man, "I was left behind many years ago. I was without a home and belonged nowhere for a very long time. So, I kept on pursuing and searching for where I belonged over the years. Hoping to reunite and once again prevail together through this life. Regrettably, I thought I would never find that again. Or perhaps to put it in a better tense, who I was looking for would never find me. That was until the other day, when I saw you at the base of the dark side of the mountain. As we began our course up the mountain together, I had asked you not to speak of anything about doubt, negativity, or fear until we made it to our final destination. As we continued towards the unknown, we began to bond through motion, which in turn caused emotion. The more dangerous the climb, the more engaged we had become. With every small triumph, we became more powerful in thought and emotion. Our confidence flourished with every step. As we got to the top of the goliath, we became unbreakable. I could see my new home facing in front of me. For the unknown is where I belong. Amid the known, I was forgotten. Laid to rest. Being completely overshadowed by doubt, comparison, judgement, ambiguity, disbelief, habit, blame, complacency, apprehension, jealousy and most predominantly fear. I had been as big as this mountain range and could fly as high as the sun when I was believed in. Sadly, in yours and so many countless others, I was slowly forgotten as you grew older. As you experienced what was perceived as failure and conformity, you pushed me further away. Every time you have given up instead of going for it with all that you are. When you succumbed to this and made it your behaviors and habits, you had totally lost all contact with me. But I was always there, waiting and believing that I would once again be found. On this day, I was rewarded for my unwillingness to give up. You see, you named me Courage when you believed in me a long time ago, when you were a child like me. But today, after all these years, in the direst of situations, with so many ways to give up, finally on the top of this mountain that we climbed together, in this serendipitous moment, finally I was reunited with where I belonged and found my way home."

THE BEES KNEES

For many years of my life, I held myself back from so many things due to my fear of failure. The true failure here is that I believed that the fear that I had created from past experiences had become the template I would conduct myself with. I would second guess everything, identify all that could potentially go wrong, predict an outcome that ended in failure, and then I would give up before even attempting to go for it. So, in essence, subconsciously, I planned to fail, not to succeed. This behavior became a habit. A habit that could evolve and adapt to any new situation, compromising growth, belief, optimism, success, and accomplishment. Why do I, and millions, if not billions of other people do this multiple times a day? To answer that, I needed to comprehend what fear is. What is it composed of? The mechanics of it. How is it created? Most importantly, where its origin stemmed from.

Fear is concocted by close mindedness to the unknown in front of you, while attempting to control the outcome by predicting it, based on past experiences.

Fear is a natural and primal human emotion. It involves a biochemical response as well as a heightened individual emotional response. Fear alerts us to the presence of danger or the potential threat of harm, whether that danger is psychological or physical. Fear can stem from real threats, but it can also originate from imagined dangers. Fear is a symptom of some mental health conditions including depression, anxiety disorder, panic disorder, phobias, and post-traumatic stress disorder (PTSD) as well as others.

Fear is composed of two primary reactions to some type of perceived threat: biochemical and emotional.

The Biochemical Response to fear is a natural emotion and a survival mechanism. When we are confronted with a perceived threat, our bodies will respond in specific consistent ways. Physical reactions to fear include a spiked increased heart rate, high adrenaline levels that make us extremely alert, sweating, trembling, or shaking, even paralysis. This is known as the "fight or flight" response. The body is preparing itself to essentially fight or to run away. I would imagine this biochemical reaction that is crucial to our survival is an instinctive evolutionary response.

The emotional response to fear can be highly personalized. Due to fear involving many of the same chemical reaction patterns in our brains that positive emotions like happiness and excitement do, sometimes feeling fear under the right circumstances can be seen as fun, like when you read a scary book, watch horror movies or when we hide and jump out scaring a friend for example.

Some people, like myself, thrive on fear-inducing thrilling

situations such as driving fast, cliff jumping, swimming with sharks, which all create an adrenaline rush. Having said that, this does not make me fearless.

The vast majority of people however have a negative reaction to the feeling of fear, which causes them to avoid fear-inducing situations at all costs. Someone who has manufactured a fear of sharks even though they have never encountered one may never step foot in the ocean, or a lake, or even a swimming pool in the darkness of night.

Although the physical reaction is constant, the experience of fear may be perceived as either positive or negative, and this is the variable. This distressing emotion provoked by dangerous situations, pain, evil or threat is the feeling of being afraid. People are afraid of a great many things and because we all were exposed to different circumstances within our environments in our lives this is why we do not all share the same fears. Therefore, whether the fear is physical or imagined as most are, the reactions are very similar. These reactions can be passed on and taught to our children, family, and friends to behave in the same manner towards a "threat" so to speak. Here are two examples of the same "threat" or constants but the reactions creating the variable outcomes in a completely different way.

When I was a little boy, I loved collecting creepy crawlers. I loved reptiles, amphibians, insects, and arachnids. The animals in which most people fear or would like to step on. On a spring or summer day I would take an emptied and cleaned out jar with a lid in which I poked many tiny little air holes in. I would sit in the middle of a massive field that was decorated with Purple Lilacs, Yellow Evening Primrose, Milkweed, Giant Hyssops, Yellow clovers, Dandelions and so many other flowering plants, weeds, and shrubs. Huge patches of dusty pink and white alsike clovers filled the air with their sweet comforting scent. Sometimes even the occasional Prairie Rose, a stunning pink flower found on the ground. I would find a spot that had a lot of activity with bees. Huge fat bumble bees everywhere. Honeybees, even though an invasive species, are the most common bee buzzing around in any direction that I looked. Some of the other two hundred plus species of bees that inhabit Manitoba, made appearances as well. Dragon flies in magnificent iridescent armor highlighted with bright green, turquoise and yellow stripes took rest on many of the flowers. Always beautiful butterflies including my favorite, the Monarch were gracefully floating and flying from flower to flower. A true gift from nature was when Ruby Throated Hummingbirds would fly into the area while I was observing the ecosystems of pollination. An astonishing and fairly frequent sighting back then. Unfortunately, not anymore, as these areas are now populated by strip malls, apartment buildings, condominiums, and developments of Lego like houses packed so closely together.

When I saw a bee doing its thing on a flower, I would slowly surround it with the jar and then close the lid on the flower gently encouraging the bee to fly inside the jar. From there I would study and observe the bee up close. I began to learn the different characterizations of each species of bee. The bees generally were not aggressive while in my captivity at all. After a minute or so once the bee had relaxed somewhat, I gave it a name and I opened the lid, and the bee flew away when it was ready to travel to another area of flowers. I would do this for hours never once being stung by a bee. I had previously been attacked on my face causing severe swelling and bruising by multiple Yellow Jacket Wasps, when I mistakenly ripped open their nest inside a thick shrub when picking Saskatoon berries with my grandmother near Winnipeg Beach. It was incredibly painful, frightening at first, yet I had no fear of bees when I returned to the open grass areas I frequented. In fact, I began to handle the bees with my bare hands, butterflies would land on my head, face and shoulders as did Dragonflies. For me this was remarkable and thrilling. In my mind I had become one with the animals within that ecosystem. I felt like I was Tarzan and that was my jungle.

In the present when I see a bee, which sadly has dramatically diminished in occurrence, I have no fear of it and my behavior dictates calmness and can become contagious with people around me. I often share some of the knowledge that I have regarding bees in that situation which is generally positively received. Well, by some of them.

On the other hand, when many people see a bee, their reaction is the polar opposite of mine. I have personally witnessed throughout my life hundreds of people from all different walks of life become paralyzed with fear or run away screaming from a bee flying close by.

Both of my sisters were both terrified of bees. They reacted in the way I described above. Neither of them has been stung by a bee. Their environments that they grew up in were very different, yet the exact same reaction. Of course, there is an instinctive fear of being stung by a bee as it can be very painful and that is scary. One of our brain's main functions is to preserve our life in the safest way possible. Through thousands of years' worth of imprinted DNA our brain has become hard wired in this process. But I believe that there is more to it than just that. I believe that the fear of bees is manufactured in our young minds as children. We take in all the information given to us as our brain collects everything to learn how to live.

At a young age we watch how our parents, relatives and friends behave and that shapes our direction of personal growth, or the lack thereof. I think that as a very young child the individual was exposed to a behavior regarding bees. Perhaps they watched their parents react in horror as a bee approached. Maybe one of them ran away muttering swear words you had never heard before. Perhaps they swooped you up and saved your life from that menacing killer bee. As these overreactions continue it solidifies as a habit. The young mind absorbs this as regular behavior over time regarding when coming in the proximity of a bee. We teach fear to our children by default. Now as they get older and see a bee their reaction is the same as the one, they were exposed to by a symbol of trust, such as their parents. The child inherits the behavior and forms the same reactive habits. In essence, the fear we do not face becomes our limits. A taught fear that is all perception and the fear widely created in our minds as people predict the worst-case scenario when faced with that fear. We are presented with the same constant, being the bee, and the variable being the reaction to the bee.

This supports my belief that we are taught fear by the important people around us as we grow up. This continues through school as well. As children we start to feel different or separated from other kids based on social structures in place in the classroom. We watch as some kids are very intelligent, some become good at sports, others good at both. But this is all based on comparison to the performance of the other kids. Even though the students have completely different upbringings, schools expect the same results for everyone. This created a divide within the group and social fear, or anxiety was born. I could never keep up with the other kids academically and I started to feel like a failure because of this. It became embarrassing and humiliating for me and with the social pressures of the classroom my fear of failure was created. Self-defeating thoughts took over my mind and eventually I would just not do what I was supposed to do because I predicted failure as the outcome before it even happened. I attached that manufactured fear to the emotion of a result from a past circumstance. Predicting the future by using the past. This grew with me throughout my life to the point that I rarely believed in myself enough to even bother trying. Or if I was becoming successful with something I would sabotage my opportunity by being afraid of succeeding because I did not believe that I deserved it, due to the hardwiring of my brain. I also did not know how to feel that. So, I feared it.

Fear causes hesitation and hesitation causes our fear to come true.

Most of us were utterly fearless as children. We climbed trees, jumped off things, dove into the deep end, slid down slides face first, picked up snakes and so on and so on. We followed our imagination, not our analytics. Because there wasn't an experience previously to tell our brain otherwise. Now of course if an adult saw their child halfway up a tree, they would exercise caution and most likely say to come down from up there, you could fall and hurt yourself. Reluctantly we climbed down most times and going forward we began to analyze the potential to fall and get hurt, hindering the height of our climb.

We carry this with us throughout our lives, in relationships, work, goals and dreams. Focusing on the safety of what could go wrong versus what could go right.

Here is a perfect example of that. I have asked many people over the years what was their most significant memory as a young child. The answer most times was riding a bicycle for the very first time by themselves. Without the aid of training wheels or an adult. The same goes for me. The reason that this is such a powerful memory is due to it being the first time in my cognitive development that I did not hesitate and give in to fear. Many prior attempts before, my father would hold the bike and run beside me telling me just to pedal. And would then tell me that he was about to let go of me. Because I was concentrating on him letting go of me, I began to create the fear of what if I fell, got hurt, would people laugh at me, essentially all that could go wrong. As soon as my dad let go of me, I wiped out. The fear that I predicted came true. Scraping up my knees, chin, elbows, shins, and some bruises were common. I would break down in frustration and get angry or sometimes cry because I failed. My dad would simply tell me to get back on the bike and give it another try again.

Finally, one day we were out in the bay and my dad was again running beside me holding the bike steady so I would not fall, he told me to keep pedaling, so I did. This time my dad let go of me and didn't tell me. Instead of the projected fear I would normally feel because of him telling me when he was letting go, this time I had no hesitation. Therefore, no fear. I rode that bike around my bay as many times as I could. My dad cheered me on! I felt so alive. In my mind it felt like I was flying a rocket ship at the speed of light down the road because I was going so fast. The smile on my face was bigger than the entire world at that moment. Unfortunately, I was not taught how to stop by using the brakes on the bike. So, as I attempted to slow down, I breezed past my dad as he was yelling "use the brakes, use the brakes!" and I coasted right into the back end of a parked car on a driveway a few houses down sending me flying off the bike landing on the pavement scraping and reopening cuts on my knees. I got up, felt no pain whatsoever. I looked at my dad and asked if I could ride it again, so I did. Over and over again. Thankfully, I also learned how to use the brakes to stop which was better than crashing into large solid stationary objects in order to do so.

The significance of this moment is this. It was the first time that fear did not cause hesitation. Alternatively, I just did it without any fear. When we hesitate, we over think, complicate, over analyze what we are doing. This hesitation causes the fear to come true. Why? Because we are focused on creating the worst possible outcome and then it materializes in that exact moment. We create fear, we create the outcome. Throughout life, people will talk themselves out of doing something they really want by creating the fear of failing before even attempting it. Sadly, this is commonly based on two things. What will people think? What will people say? Those are the two biggest killers of actions, goals, ambitions, and dreams. I, like many, because of those two killers, choose our path out of fear disguised as practicality and conformity. We conform to what we are taught to believe is the safe and sound way of being just like everyone else. We are taught not to stand out by our personalities but instead by our accomplishments. Our individualism is judged and because of that it is sadly often molded into a lackluster version of its true self. We are subjected to constant comparison in all our social habitats throughout our lives. At home, school, sports, religious or spiritual places, workplace and all the relationships within them.

Fear is always about what does not exist, we create it and give it meaning, power and life. But it still does not exist. We give it life because we are attempting to control something we don't understand but end up altering our behavior for it. Fear is a projection of an outcome based on feelings from experiences that we manufacture in our own minds. It is an illusion.

Therefore, fear does not exist when we replace it with courage. Courage is the demise of fear.

How to deal with fear. Stop creating it. Write that down.

CHAPTER 8

THE BEST FISH TACOS IN MEXICO

The secret to doing anything is believing that you can do it. Anything that you believe you can do strong enough, you can do. Anything. As long as you believe.
Bob Ross

I have been visiting Mexico every year, sometimes twice a year for over a decade. Basically, whenever I could. I fell in love with the Riviera Maya. It is the stretch of Caribbean coastline along the Yucatan Peninsula. Cancun being the main hub of tourism. A big city with hotels and resorts along the ocean and the lagoon side as well. A fun place to party with truly mind-blowing night clubs. A bit south is Puerto Morales, a beautiful and quaint fishing town located south of Cancun with its charming restaurants. Further down is Playa Del Carmen with its incredible Resorts accompanied with a great city headlined by 5th avenue. Bars, restaurants, shopping, and everything else you can imagine. Endless stretches of white powder like sands melting into the captivating crystal-clear turquoise waters of the Caribbean Ocean. Directly across the ocean is the intoxicating island of Cozumel. The best place to swim with giant and gentle Whale Sharks during the summer months. A quick forty-five-minute ferry ride from Playa Del Carmen. A vibrant and chill community with exceptional snorkeling and scuba diving spots located on reefs just off the island. Even further south along the main coastline are the towns of Akumal and Tulum. Akumal, which means "land of the turtle" in Mayan, has endless beaches and coral reefs that are home to many species of wildlife including Green Sea Turtles. Tulum, a nearby town just down the coastline of the Caribbean Ocean has ancient Mayan ruins close by and cenotes to explore.

I often found myself wandering the streets in these small Mexican towns off the Caribbean Ocean. Not on the resort property, not on a big fancy lit up street with bars and stores. Just streets with small markets, houses, decorations, and the people that lived there. I was always in search of a taco stand where I could buy fish tacos with fresh fish, caught that day from the ocean and to wash it down with a cold Mexican cerveza. Oceanside was always preferable. I enjoyed meeting people and attempting to communicate with my horribly embarrassing attempts at speaking Mexican Spanish. Luckily for me, most of the locals I met spoke better broken English and because of that we were able to hold conversations. I would show them pictures on my phone and tell them about the stories behind them. We shared lots of laughs and lots at my expense but worth it to see their faces light up. Developing new connections while bridging the communication gap which was beautifully organic in its nature.

One day in 2010, everything changed when I met a younger boy named Juan.

I had wandered in a different direction that day after leaving the comforts of my resort. I liked being out before anyone else and was walking the beach for about an hour after my early morning workout. It was a sunny hot day with a very gentle calm breeze that was just cool enough to be refreshing on the moisture of sweat of my skin. The sky was decorated with thin strips of white cirrus clouds that looked like they were put there by paint brush strokes. Every fifteen or twenty minutes when I got too hot, I would run and plunge into the perfect picture of what an ocean view looked like, to cool myself down. The water was an iridescent turquoise blue and felt like silk as I swam through it. It was the perfect temperature. Diving into oncoming waves and then turning around and body surfing the next wave back in. I was in waist deep water but when the waves passed the water became chest deep. I was surrounded by a small school of about thirty to forty shiny silver fish that were marked with yellow and black stripes known as Sergeant Majors. A very common reef fish from that area about the size of a small dinner plate. They were all swimming in synchronicity around me. It was hypnotically mesmerizing to watch them move through the water together. They had no fear of me as I stood there motionless. As though they were putting on an underwater show for me. Then, suddenly without warning, all the fish got spooked by something and took off in a flash, heading for the shallower water straight ahead. It was right then when I could feel a presence behind me in the water and just as I turned my head over my shoulder to the left of me, I could see a large dark shadow approaching in the wave that was oncoming a meter behind me. That moment turned into slow motion as the water swelled while the wave passed by. The shadow turned to bright silver as the wave exposed the fish into the sunlight beside me. It was a Great Barracuda. A very large predatory fish shaped like a cylindrical missile with dark blotches and bands down its side. Its large, pointed head was made up primarily of powerful jaws that housed rows of razor-sharp conical teeth about half the size of my thumb used to eat its prey. Massive black eyes that were quite fearsome in appearance. As this magnificent creature glided inside the wave only a foot away from me, its eyes locked on mine. Everything stopped in the world except for what was happening at that perfect moment where primordial instinctive fear and breathtaking excitement had merged into the same feeling. The barracuda was about five feet long. I would guess that it weighed over sixty pounds of solid predatory muscle. As both of our eyes locked for what seemed like forever, I wondered what that beautiful wild animal was thinking.? Did it consider me to be a threat to its environment? Or another predator competing in its hunting territory? Or did it think what is this stupid clumsy human doing in my backyard? As it passed me, its ink black eyes shifted another direction and then like a flash of lightning it exploded into the shallower waters. Darting at its prey just two meters ahead of me. As quick as it attacked the fish in front of me, it then disappeared back into the deeper waters behind me. It was an experience like no other I had felt before. It was electrifying. It took me a few minutes to process all of it. Thinking to myself what a miracle I had just been witness to. To see such a rare phenomenon like that was such an undeniable blessing from Mother Nature.

As I made my way back to the beach and returned to the sugar like powder sands. My attention shifted. I could hear someone yelling off in the distance. I looked over to see what appeared to be a younger boy struggling with a fishing rod on the shore about a hundred feet down the beach. I was not sure if he was yelling at me or for help, but I took off running towards him. As I approached, I could see he had a big plastic tub full of a few different species of fish and was currently battling another fish on his line. The young boy who I guessed was probably around twelve years old, looked at me and very enthusiastically said "Hey! Johnny Bravo! Do you like fish tacos?!" I was a bit caught off guard by his English and his questions. I laughed and said, "I love fish tacos!" The boy asked me, "Do you want to eat the best fish tacos in Mexico, Johnny Bravo?" Ci amigo. I responded. I helped him reel in one last large fish and placed it in the container with the others. He muttered something in Mexican to the fish and then looked at me and smiled while flexing his biceps for me to acknowledge. He motioned for me to do the same. I obliged. It appeared as though we were having a Mexican standoff, guns blazing during the gun show on the beach. We both laughed. He told me that the fish he just caught was for making tacos for lunch and dinner. He made a comment about how big my muscles were and then motioned for me to carry the tub of fish for him, putting my muscles to work. I shrugged and smiled and picked up the container and started following the kid towards a path that cut through the shrubs and trees on the edge where the jungle met the beach. He told me his name was Juan. That his family made the best tacos in Mexico. I told him my name was Jay and I was excited to try them. As the winding path opened to the road, he asked me where I was from. I told him from Winnipeg, a city at the heart of the country Canada. He told me that he had met many people from Canada and that they were all good people. Always nice to hear. He told me that he had always lived there. We walked to the roadside, where he motioned for me to put the container of fish down. He explained to me his older brother would be there soon to pick him up. He asked what resort I was staying at, and I told him which one. Looking at me he said that he would be out front of the resort at lunchtime and for me to come meet him there so he could introduce me to the best fish tacos in Mexico. Sounded like a plan to me. As I began to walk away, Juan yelled "Hey!" and as I turned around, he was nodding his head smiling while flexing his biceps at me and laughingly said "Johnny Bravo!"

I laughed and waved back to him. I can remember feeling so full of life from that morning. I made my way back up the beach to my resort. It was getting very hot in the sun. Just before noon that day, I walked through the lush grounds of the resort, its mazes of swimming pools and bars, through the huge open lobby made of marble accents with giant statues. As I made my way to the security station at the entrance to the resort, I was met by staff asking me where I was going. After a brief conversation I exited the property and there was Juan waiting for me. He greeted me with excitement and said we had a ten-minute walk to his taco stand. As we walked, I asked him how he learned to speak English so well. He explained that he had always been a fast learner. He wanted to learn because it was important to be able to tell tourists about his family's business. Mission accomplished. We entered a small village like town. Quaint surroundings with traditional Mexican flare to it. As we walked past people Juan always had something to say that made them laugh. When we arrived at his taco stand, I was greeted by some of his family. There were a few locals having lunch, sitting on the colorful plastic chairs nearby. I attempted to order some fish tacos speaking in Spanish but was met with looks of humored confusion. Juan piped in and said that I wanted four tacos. His father smiled as he manned the grill and his mother prepared the homemade tortilla with lettuce, Pico de Gallo, a family secret recipe taco sauce that had a hint of lime and finally cilantro sprinkled over top. The fresh fish was buttery in texture and cooked perfectly. I grabbed a cold bottle of Pacifico from the cooler and sat down and ate all four of my deliciously mouthwatering tacos. Juan watched me with intensity waiting for my response. I yelled out "the best fish tacos in Mexico!!!!" Everyone nearby stopped talking and stared at me for a second. As if cued by a maestro, they all burst into laughter like a symphony. A truly beautiful moment where language did not really matter. The rawness of emotion was our tool of communication. Juan sat with me for a bit, and he asked me to see pictures on my phone of where I lived. A few of the other kids gathered around as well and I showed them some photos of my life. I showed them Facebook on my phone as well. They were intrigued by all the pictures and people that shared them on my feed. After I finished my lunch, I walked through the small town and bought a few things at the tiny market there. I told Juan that I would be back the next day for more tacos. Throughout the remainder of the day, I reflected on the magical experience that took place. How the unique connection between the occurrences that happened that morning was a statement from the universe that everything happens for a reason without coincidence. I chose to walk a different path that morning which led me to the spot in the ocean where I encountered the Great Barracuda, which was at the same time as Juan was fishing in the ocean a hundred feet away. Hearing his call and deciding to go investigate the situation. That investigation introduced me to Juan. Juan with his charismatic and humorous character convinced me to meet up with him to eat the best fish tacos in Mexico. Which I did. Thank you, Universe!

The next day around lunchtime, I made my way back to Juan's family taco stand. I tried a different type of fish this time in my tacos, but it was just as good as the previous ones the day before. It was the special sauce and oil used to fry the fish. Juan was ecstatic to see me. We sat and chatted for a while. Juan asked me to see Facebook again. He was scrolling through my feed and stopped on a post. I could see a very concerned and contemplative look on the little guy's face. Juan asked me why this person was complaining that their car wouldn't start. I looked at him and smiled and I told him that some people that are unhappy like to post about it, so they can find other people that aren't happy, and they can be unhappy together and they would complain about everything and whine all day long. I explained to him that it is called a pity party. He told me he would never attend that kind of party, that it sounded like an awful party. The young boy looked at me and I could see that he was deep in thought and then he said to me why would anybody post that kind of stuff when they could be reaching out to their family, telling them that they love them. He also said that he could maybe try to find some of his older brothers to tell them that he misses him, and he is alive and well. He went on to tell me that he would post stories about his family's history and his country's dedication to preserving its natural ecology. He would like to share the Day of the Dead celebration and post beautiful pictures of the incredible parade that happens in his hometown every year. Capturing all the amazing costumes and people in the streets.

It hit me right there and then like a punch between the eyes, the difference between his world and mine. It became quite apparent in that moment how embarrassing the self-centered entitlement that existed in my world. Everyday people complain about everything. Going on rants about how someone at a fast-food place made a mistake on their order and that they recommended you never go there ever! Don't get me wrong, there are people that post beautiful pictures and positive inspirational and motivational posts, but for the greater majority at that time it had become an artificial virtual pity party.

The little Mexican boy named Juan had never seen anything else other than the place that he lived. He told me he had dreams of seeing the whole world. I showed him on my phone pictures and videos of every country he asked about. His face lit up colorfully bright like light coming through stained glass. He was so excited and wanted to find out more. He had three brothers and two sisters but hadn't seen his two oldest brothers in a year. He then asked me if I could help him find them. Curiously I asked Juan. How could I do that? He looked up at me with a contagiously hopeful smile and said, "Johnny Bravo, what if you put a picture of me on your Facebook with a message for my brothers? If everybody is connected to the internet, maybe someone will see my picture who knows my brothers, or maybe his brothers will see his picture and happily reply to it. I thought to myself what a beautiful, genuine, hopeful, and faithful young man. I could see in his eyes that he truly believed that there was a possibility for this to work. I told him that he was brilliant, and it was an awesome idea! So, I took a couple pictures of little Juan. I was so excited to post his picture. He told me that his brothers did not speak English, so he would like to write his message in Spanish Mexican. So, he did. And then I posted it. Juan was so full of electricity and excitement and hope that he asked me if anyone had responded only a minute later. I laughed and said, "I'm sorry, my new friend, not yet." However, I started to receive a lot of comments and questions from various people that saw this post on my page. They asked what was going on in this picture? Did I adopt a Mexican child? Where in Mexico was this picture taken? Did you make new friends down there? I replied explaining about Juan's idea and message and that was met with so much pessimism. "There's no way that will ever happen." that's impossible" and then I replied that Juan believes that it will happen and at the Impossible can be done. Juan asked me what the people on my feed were saying? I looked at him and I smiled and said they all want to help you find your brothers and they're going to do whatever they can to help you. He rubbed his hands together with excitement. He had the biggest smile on his face that beamed brighter than the sunshine and he started jumping up and down. There's no way I would ever tell him the ugly truth as it was disturbing and disgusting. Negative and disheartening. I guess it just really made me realize how far off course we had come. How spoiled rotten we were. Taking so many things for granted, mocking the power of belief, and how negative and cynical my world and the people in it had become.

I visited Juan and his family every day, eating their fish tacos and drinking their cervezas for the remainder of my time there. I would spend an hour or two around lunch and then sometimes return for an hour at dinner time. Every day we checked his post to see if his brothers had seen it and every day, had to tell him not yet, but they will if you continue to believe. The last day before I caught my flight home, I told Juan that I would be back next year at the same time. I told him by that time your brother's will have found you and you will be reunited one day. We're both sad to see each other go our separate ways. I told him I would come find him at his taco stand the next time I was there, and I wanted some free tacos. I said goodbye to his family and as I walked back to the resort I began to tear up. The realization that a little kid that had nothing believed in everything. While the people I knew had everything but believed in nothing.

When I returned home, I kept the post up and then continued to re-post it a couple times. Some people thought the post was a very cute idea, some thought I was doing it to make myself look better, but sadly most people laughed at a one in a billion chance it would ever happen. Months and months went by, and Juan and I had exchanged addresses so we could mail each other letters, as he did not have access to email, or the internet for that matter. Every letter he wrote asked me if his brothers saw the post. Each time I would write back and have to tell him the disappointing news, not yet, but don't give up hope. We wrote each about once every few weeks for about eleven months. Then unexpectedly, I didn't hear back from Juan, so I wrote him another letter and mailed it to him. Again, without a response or reply. I was concerned but was also hoping for the best for him. I would be back in Mexico in less than a month's time and thought maybe that's why he had not replied. Perhaps he was just awaiting my arrival.

The following month I returned to the same Mexican town and resort. Arriving later in the evening, I couldn't wait to go find and surprise Juan and his family at their Taco Stand. I got up early the morning after my arrival. The sun was just coming up. I ran along the endless beach as the waves crashed from the beautiful ocean melodically with my stride. I was hoping to find Juan fishing near the same spot but to my dismay, he was nowhere to be found. I went back to the resort where I was staying and showered. For breakfast I ate delicious fresh fruits and crepes drenched in caramel sauce. I enjoyed an espresso as I took in the warm winds that caressed my face in the open eating area facing the ocean. Reminding me of why I had an eternal love affair with this tropical paradise. I spent about half an hour swimming in the ocean and then relaxing on the beach for a couple hours. It was nearing lunch time and it was time for me to go to Juan's family taco stand. When I arrived, his father had a big smile and gave me a hug welcoming me with a boisterous "Johnny Bravo!" His mother said the same thing, a couple of the other kids clapping happily to see me. I asked where Juan was. Juan's mother smiled at me and made a gesture with her hand as to say one minute and went inside. When she came out there was no sign of Juan. Instead, she handed me an envelope and then held her hands like she was praying. There were tears slowly running down her face. I thought the worst to myself. I thought that something had happened to Juan, and he was gone. I nervously opened the envelope and inside it I found a folded piece of paper which Juan had written on. It said Johnny Bravo when you get this letter, I'm sorry that I'm not there to thank you in person. He explained that his brothers came home, and they had all been finally reunited. He went off to work in a tobacco farm for a couple months in the Mexican State of Nayarit with his two older brothers. Juan told me he would write to me again once he was back home and tell me all about his adventures with his older brothers. Juan finished his letter by saying this: the message that we sent out on Facebook had brought his brothers home, back to his family. He believed that because we put it out there, it had caused a ripple effect within the universe and that is how his brothers came home. That if you believe with everything that you are that anything is possible, it will eventually happen. Just like he believed that I would return to visit and that's why he hadn't chosen to write to me and tell me the news. That instead, he knew I would come there and to prove it, is why he left the letter behind with his family. He closed the letter out with this "of course you can have a free taco, every time you buy four tacos, you get a free one Senor Johnny Bravo."

I laughed out loud after I read that. Saying to myself you little rascal. It was in that pure moment that I had a revelation. You see, I thought I had taught Juan so much in the short time while I was there. But in actuality, it was Juan who taught me so much more in the time it took me to read his letter. The fisherman's son who had never seen a smartphone, the internet or anywhere else in the world other than the small beach town that he lived in. The teen age boy who learned English on his own so he could promote to tourists that he had the best fish tacos in all of Mexico and would be able to converse with them. That he and his family who lived in a tiny two-bedroom house that was partially made of just plywood, that our spoiled rotten sense of entitlement and self-righteous standards of society would look down upon as poverty like conditions, were unconditionally happy and thankful for what they had. Most importantly Juan taught me three things that I would not truly understand until years later. The power of hope, the power of belief and the power of purpose. Which were all such lacking factors in my life that contributed to the damage of the state of my mental health. The combination of these three fundamentals were far more valuable than all the materialistic things I thought I had built into my identity to compensate for my unhappiness. The teacher graciously became the student right there in that moment which has stuck with me over the course of my time.

Whether or not the post on my Facebook truly did reach his brothers I will never know. But somehow, deep down I believe that it did. Perhaps through conversation and thought that it transcended on a different level of communication. One of manifestation, due to belief that it would. I will never know the truth of all of this. However, Juan's belief system had a ripple effect on me which caused me to believe enough to share his story with the optimistic intent of strengthening your hope, belief and finding purpose in your life like it unambiguously did in mine. Without belief, a miracle does not exist.

Side note: They were absolutely the best fish tacos I have eaten in my travels throughout my life and have been back there many times. Juan is now a young man and a father of a beautiful family. So, if you are in Caribbean side of Mexico, I strongly suggest you try them. But you will have to find them on your own just like I did. I cannot tell you exactly where because that is the best part of the adventure. But I will say this, Akumal is one the most beautiful places in the world and one my personal favorites. The resorts along the ocean are exceptional and the small quaint town is close by and awaiting your discovery. White sand beaches melt into clear turquoise ocean water with bountiful coral reefs where you can snorkel with sea turtles, rays, and many other different diverse and colorful species of fish. There is an abundance of eco parks and animal sanctuaries in the jungle to discover and explore within the proximity. I am happy to report that there are many species of frogs in the lush tropical ecosystems in the surrounding area. Ride bicycles, sail on boats, chase waves in kayaks all in the same day. The Mayan ruins nearby connect the soul with rich traditional Mexican heritage while walking on paths winding through the ancient architecture from civilizations nearly a thousand years old. I personally recommend getting up early and walking the beach, there you will find all kinds of people fishing as the sun rises. Fascinating people to talk to. You just never know where a conversation may take you...guiño guiño.

CHAPTER 9

STICKS AND STONES

Don't speak negatively about yourself, even as a joke. Your body doesn't know the difference. Words are energy and cast spells. That's why it's called spelling. Change the way you speak about yourself, and you can change your life. What you're not changing, you're also choosing.
Bruce Lee

I wasn't happy with myself because I truly didn't know myself. I was depressed because I knew I was not doing what would make me happy in life. I had never taken the time to understand who I was and why I was like the way I was. Which led to a very dysfunctional relationship with myself. I feel as though this is the common denominator among many people who are feeling loneliness, worthless, empty, powerless, flawed, inadequate, desperate, disheartened, unhappiness, desolate and angry due to depression. This is based on what I felt. I talked with as many people as I could to understand a broader perspective of what depression felt like to them or what they imagined depression felt like. When I explained to a few close friends that these were the states of feeling I was so used to and that from the moment I woke up I was met with self-discouragement, self-hate, disgrace, the list goes on and on. Some days I just felt like I had nothing left, I had written myself off. My inner dialogue had become one of the key components in my defeated state. I would wake up and begin my day by telling myself that there was no point to anything in my life, I was a waste of life, that I didn't deserve to live, I had nothing left to give to anyone, I wasn't strong enough to go on, and this led to my suicidal ideation taking off like a wildfire. It went from thinking about it a couple times a week to daily and then to hourly. I had become obsessed with taking my life. My inner dialogue was like something I wouldn't have ever said to another human being. That is when I articulately and strategically began developing the timeline of when I would take my life. I stopped talking to most people that called or messaged me. I didn't visit with my family. When and if I was at work my co-workers could tell something was not right, drastic changes in my behavior and demeanor. I looked exhausted. I was no longer quick witted with my outrageous sense of humor. A dull burnt-out light. I would constantly make references to killing myself disguised as jokes. I was not joking at all. I was as serious as a heart attack.

The age old saying "sticks and stones may break my bones, but names will never hurt me" is in fact misleading. Yes, sticks and stones could possibly break bones in a variety of circumstances. However, the statement of "names will never hurt me" is where I disagree. As we grow through life there are certain "names" we have been called by others that stick to us like glue. Over that course of time, internalization of that name and its connotations becomes the fabric that holds us in association with it. An example would be if I saw someone from my past and they had called me names and made fun of me when I was a young teenager, I would immediately revert to the associated feelings that occurred so many years ago. Then recalibrating my emotional present projection of that person through an internal collective. Through years of bullying this could cause imminent anger and discomfort towards that person immediately. I had to ask myself Why? It was because I held on to the emotional attachment of that feeling, extending its damage to myself by carrying it throughout my life. Altering a self-conscious reaction anytime I heard someone else say something similar. Essentially victimizing myself and holding on to it like a form of self-punishment. Meanwhile, the person who insulted me years ago has moved on and not even given it a single thought since. They could care less and most likely have zero recollection of the insulting event ever taking place. I had to teach myself how to let go of these self-induced punishments by simply writing down the insult and breaking it down to the core. Once I was able to pinpoint the reason why it had bothered me, I was able to see how ridiculous it was and usually laugh it off. Exposing an opportunity to interpret more about myself and why the name or insult had taken an effect on me and to let it be and no longer allow it to take up valuable residence in my mind.

Another example which holds tremendously more damaging repercussions were the names I would assign to myself and negative things I would say to myself. Since I was a little boy, I have always called myself stupid, telling myself that I would always be stupid and perpetually always do stupid things. What I was inadvertently doing was creating the engineering instructions for my brain to begin hardwiring this into a blueprint. The more I insulted myself, the more it became a permanent imprint in my pathological programming. Essentially empowering limitations. Over time becoming a default habitual reactive reminder to myself when I was having difficulty understanding something. This would be forged into a behavior cueing an action to do something stupid afterwards such as act out or overreact while synchronously insulting myself more. Sadly, this would become part of my identity or what I would identify myself as to myself.

Subsequently, I would subconsciously then project that upon myself anytime I was faced with any intellectual adversity because now it had been fully hardwired into my brain functioning. This would set off the precursory stages of a chain reaction that anytime I had a new opportunity to learn or grow I would subconsciously prepare myself to fail and sabotage the opportunity before I even gave it a shot, impeding development and growth of my mind because I was too afraid of looking stupid. This would set off more reactions such as the emotions of shame and guilt that would trigger more negative internal dialogue battering myself down with more unforgiving insults and harsh self judgement. Creating a catastrophic downward spiral of self-doubt taking away the ability to believe in myself, leaving me feeling worthless. This emotionality cycle would continue to intensify. As a result, these compounded reactions would create self-destructive behaviors I would carry with me for most of my life.

On the contrary side of things, When I would talk positively to myself and not complain about myself or my situation, the opposite compounding reactions would then present themselves. When my verbiage changed when I talked to myself in my mind or at times out loud, to an optimistic viewpoint, I felt happier. I would not insult or lay down any infringing titles upon myself. Encouraging and empowering myself to move forward regardless of the obstacles attempting to prohibit my progression. This would set off more positive chemical reactions inside my brain that would contribute to mood stabilization, esteem, and overall greater production due to increased energy. Challenging my brain to expand. Firing millions upon millions of neurons into a new connection frenzy. Producing indisputable and decisive onward momentum.

I had to ask myself how my inner dialogue dictates the positive or negative inertia of momentum. To illustrate this, imagine two identical mountains side by side with each other. Halfway to the top of each mountain there is an immense accumulation of water the size of a small lake created by rainfall and water making its way down from the peaks of each mountain. Both are equal in size and mass. When envisioning the mountains, the first mountain is called Negatron and the mass of the lake is made up of water molecules that will be composed of negative thoughts, feelings, and emotions. The other mountain is called Optimistic Prime, and its identical amount of water molecules are composed of positive thoughts, feelings, and emotions.

When I think of negative thoughts which initiate negative feelings and emotions, I generally feel a cumbersome weight upon myself. Negative thoughts are hard on the mind and body which cause negative feelings mentally and physically, which then cause negative emotions like sadness, fear, or anger. Physically causing negative states like lack of energy and unproductivity. This is when internal dialogue turns very negative towards ourselves adding to the lumbering load. Negativity tends to hold people down with its cumulative weight. Negative momentum.

On the contrary, positive thoughts generate positive feelings and emotions which have truly the opposite effect. When I think of positive things, I feel lighter. Positive feelings are healthy for both the mind and body creating a state of harmonious productivity. These feelings cause positive emotions such as happiness. The more positive things we think or feel, the more likely we will remain in a positive state. States like freedom, creativity, and bliss. When positive inner dialogue takes place, the more positive and uplifted we become. Positivity as in a mindset tends to free people and help them move forward in life. We feel lighter. Positive momentum.

Following this model based on thoughts, feelings and emotions, the negative water molecules are substantially heavier than the positive water molecules. Exactly the same number of molecules in the identical mass of each body of water upon the twin mountains.

A shift in a tectonic plate causes both mountains to shake and vibrate considerably at the same rate, causing an equal size crack to form at the top of each mountain. The lakes on each of the mountains are affected by the vibrations as well which creates a ripple effect of energy through the water. The energy travels from the back of the lakes, and then all the way to the front. This causes a wave to form on each lake, however, because the negative water molecules are heavier, the wave on top of Negatron picks up more velocity and creates a more powerful force. As it reaches the newly formed crack on the mountain water begins to push its way through it. Due to the energy and power of the wave its pressure on the crack is tremendous and suddenly after a few drops of water make their way through the crack, the entire mass begins to push through as well, becoming overbearing. A massive amount of water smashes its way through instantly creating a flash flood recklessly spilling over the mountain side. Uncontrollably rushing down the mountain creating land and mudslides everywhere it touches. The Juggernaut picks up more damaging energy as the flood destroys everything in its path. Killing plants, animals, uprooting forests as it continues its destructive path down the mountain. The flood swallows up dirt, sand, rocks, trees, adding additional mass to its out-of-control runaway train like velocity. The more it destroys, the more powerful it becomes. Leaving a path of reckless devastation behind it. Eventually the sheer mass of the negative energy completely wipes out the entire mountain side. Changing the complexion to one that is now unrecognizable. Ecosystems and habitats are annihilated in the process. When the flood finally begins to lose its inertia and all the extra debris like tree trunks and boulders that were picked up begins forming blockades, the water runs its course until there is nothing or nowhere left to go. As fast as it happened, it's all over. Leaving only decimation and carnage behind.

Concurrently, the wave on the other mountain Optimistic Prime begins to reach the newly formed crack. The pressure of the wave and water composed of positive thoughts, feelings and emotions is remarkably less forceful as it finds its way into the crack. As water fills up this void, because it's lighter in composition it does not destroy its surroundings. Instead, one drop of water slowly makes its way through and falls out of the opening and then gently lands and begins to cascade down the mountainside. Another drop and then another, follow suit. These positive drops of water slowly begin to accumulate together and form a waterfall. As more water controllably finds its way through the crack it begins to slowly erode the rock and create a larger opportunity for water to flow out of it. Intensifying the waterfall. Where the waterfall meets the earth of the mountain side, streams are created. These streams with the help of gravity snake their way down the mountain following the path of least resistance. The waterfall produces a new source of unceasing water vapor that makes its way to the trees and plants below. This aids in creating new plant life and the growth and stimulus of the existing. The streams pick up sediments and carry them downward. These sediments are great carving instruments and form small pools where they are met with obstacles. The sediments enrich the soil with nutrients, making it more fertile, creating an opportunity to enhance sustainable biodiversity. Those pools provide a new habitat for all living things. New vegetation growing in the water and around the banks of the pools and ponds like plants, flowers, shrubs, and trees. Protozoans, insects, arachnids, and crustaceans make it a new home. Amphibians like frogs and salamanders sense the water source through their skin and find their way there. Fish and their eggs end up in these pools of life as well. Reptiles like turtles, lizards and snakes will find a new home here. This attracts multitudes of birds and countless small mammals. A water source for animals of all sizes to enjoy a nice drink of clean water. Housing reliable food sources for all living things. Entirely new ecosystems with so many opportunities for growth, success and new life are created down the mountain side.

If asked to choose which mountain to climb and explore between Negatron and Optimistic Prime based on the events taking place, I would pick Prime as would most other people. Optimistic Prime has an abundance of life, positive energy created by an awe-inspiring waterfall that supplements many environments. The mountain sides are stable and encouraging to explore. The chances of discovering new and exciting scenery and feeling part of its contagious energy is bountiful everywhere. Most people would be drawn to this mountain for these, and many other reasons as opposed to its counterpart Negatron. Due to its surface instability and dangerous terrain, the abundance of negative energy, destruction, and absence of life, it would be deterring too most. This is not a question of perception of the two mountains, it is a question about the reality of the connections we make to the mountains.

To take this one step further in illustrating how the way we talk to ourselves influences the direction of our momentum, imagine this.

The water that flows from the peaks of each mountain top, from rainfall to frozen glacier ice that melts into the lakes are composed of the things we say about ourselves, to ourselves, including the titles we carry and the descriptions we give ourselves. The lakes would then be our minds. The mind is filled with what comes into it by the way we talk to ourselves while experiencing situations and adversity. Negative inner dialogue creates negative thoughts which propagate negative feelings that are the genesis of negative emotional states. Positive dialogue yields the opposite results. The body of the mountains represents our mental and physical health. The living environments on the mountains serve as the environments in which we live. The crack formed on the mountain is adversity. Finally, the tectonic plate that shifts underneath the mountains is the representation of life. Life is always shifting, changing, and moving unpredictably. Producing a range of vibrations up and down the body of the mountain or in this personified case our state of mental and physical health.

In review, analyzing the events from the mountain called Negatron, the damage that the negative inner dialogue that flowed down into the mind, weighing it down with negative thoughts, feelings and emotions that are dense and heavy, cause the uncontrollable damage to mental and physical health from overflowing in an unrestrained way caused by adversity in life. Creating a rapid path of self-destruction that primarily affects itself and then secondarily everything and everyone around it in a negative way. Constituting a negative environment in the mind and body that becomes prominent in the physical environments in our lives.

Looking at the analytics of the mountain Optimistic Prime, it is plain to see it is totally the antithesis. The positive inner dialogue causes zero damage as it enters the mind. It enhances and stabilizes the mind making it more resilient to the shift of life that occurred. There was not an undisciplined overflow of overthinking or over reaction like its counterpart because the positive thoughts built positive feelings to create a sustainable positive emotional state. This allowed a focused and disciplined approach to the newly presented adversity. In turn, this shapes the waterfall of positivity that inspires growth, opportunity, and optimal health. Manufacturing a balanced mental and physical environment where the potential for success is endless while simultaneously offering itself and others a positive habitat to flourish.

I asked myself which mountain am I? For most of my life, I was Negatron. I had always talked down to myself, insulted myself and sadly by doing this I deconstructed in the ever-changing face of adversity. Shutting myself down and talking myself out of attempting many opportunities as so many others like me do. There were times when I was a combination of the two mountains as many people will be able to associate with. Generally being positive and negative except the states were controlled by the situation and scenarios put forth by life. Meaning that when life was easy and good, I was positive minded. But when life became strenuous or painful, my inner dialogue resulted negatively backwards, and I once again became Negatron. Negative words and thoughts cause the mind and body sickness. The lonely and depressed self-destructing giant.

It wasn't until after I was in isolation for a certain amount of time that I performed an autopsy on myself. Revealing and exposing how the experiences of my life had influenced either positive or negative thoughts and feelings that determined behaviors and habits. The external sources of dialogue derived from family, teachers, psychologists, friends, and kids in my early life were internalized and molded into my own inner language. Adopting a plethora of names, descriptions, and sayings that I internalized negatively about who I was. Through the process of dissecting the root of the experience that caused negative talk within and by tracing it back in time to its origin. I was able to target the source and begin to examine and eliminate all the variables and concentrate only on the constants. Patterns. Patterns of my antagonistic reactions that were hostile to myself. The abusive and traumatic circumstances that I went through had become the archetype of the constant reaction of how I would beat myself down with my inner dialogue. Reducing myself to nothing. Re-looping the damaging cycle repeatedly. The good news is that by identifying the archetype I was able to formulate a counter active strategy that enabled a positive perspective bringing light to the adverse experience as a lesson and a test of will. Removing blame, guilt and shame from the equation and replacing it with forgiveness and understanding. This would serve to teach me a new language to talk to myself with. An inner language that promoted positive adaptation and growth. This changed everything profoundly in how I viewed myself and the encompassment of my life. Like mesmerizing fireworks exploding and lighting up a warm summer night inside the dark skies of my mind. I could see everything as it could be instead of not as it couldn't be. A revelation of positive momentum.

I am now Optimistic Prime but that does not mean that it is the end of the story for Negatron. Without Negatron, Optimistic Prime cannot exist. Even with all the damages done by its creation of negative perceptions and detrimental destruction to itself. Negatron leaves behind a magnificent situation of potential to re-build, re-structure, to initiate growth, create a new life and provide a new hope. Changing the direction of momentum. Positivity is born from negativity. The positive conversations we have with ourselves when dealing with negative interference enables positive momentum. Talk to yourself like you would when helping someone you care about that's going through difficulty. Be understanding, supportive, kind, and compassionate towards yourself. Say encouraging things to yourself just like you would to someone else. By doing this I was finally able to establish a nontoxic relationship with myself. Being consistently mindful of the words I chose. I began healing. Learning to like the person I saw in the mirror as opposed to just a reflection of someone I didn't like or want to know.

It comes down to forgiveness. Think about every time a person has hurt you, lied to you, cheated you or said mean things to you. When we can simplify that the experience of them is nothing more than a thought that you hold on to and carry on. These thoughts are full of resentment, anger and dislike and are disempowering. By forgiving them through a practiced approach you release yourself from the hostile state and self-debilitating consequences like resentment. Resentment and anger are part of the venom that keeps depression and other mental illnesses or disorders running its course in our veins.

The same can be said about forgiveness when it comes to the grudges, we hold against ourselves. The times we have cheated, lied, said bad things and all the missed opportunities we hold on to punish ourselves. I personally had to learn to let these thoughts be. To leave them alone altogether. I simply did not allow them in my head after practicing self-forgiveness. Reminding myself that all the relationships I had were carried inside my head, including the one with myself. By changing the way in which I spoke to myself with positive language I was able to change what were once problems into manageable solutions in all my relationships.

The things we say and the thoughts we think are the blueprints of the house we choose to build and live in. Reminding ourselves that we will not speak to anyone else more than we speak to ourselves inside our heads, please remember to be kind

.

CHAPTER 10

LIAR, LIAR, PANTS ON FIRE

No such thing as spare time, no such thing as free time, no such thing as down time. All you got is lifetime. Go.
Henry Rollins

The truth about lying lies in the bed that we do not make in the morning, the exercise we promised ourselves we would start, the book we were going to begin reading, the habit we were going to stop doing. In order to manage disappointment with ourselves we lie to ourselves every day. The excuses that we make up are in actuality, lies. They fuel the dishonest negotiations we have with ourselves inside our heads. An excuse is a cop out. A backpedaling way out that is disregarding our personal accountability and responsibility of not acting when we need to. Excuses are made up and come to life, so we never have to go all in and take the leap of personal faith into the unknown realm of possibility. This way we think we are tricking ourselves into believing that we might act towards the desired change but deep down there will most likely be no follow through. It's like a cute cotton candy fairy tale. Robbing ourselves of the fulfilment of achievement. These lies in the form of excuses are simply manipulations of our own will and determination and all stem from our fears. Excuses are lies that we

conditionally believe because by attaching the possibility of taking action to the idea of doing something, it then makes us feel comfortable giving up before that happens. There is no change when excuses are made. In my case the more excuses I made, the more unhappy I was with myself. When the fraudulent idleness of excuse making becomes a forefront of our decision-making process especially when it comes to acting, we are providing a disservice to ourselves on so many multiple levels. Mental illness or not, self-defeating excuses hold us in the same spot hindering our momentum of movement.
Some of the most common lies disguised as sugar coated excuses regarding change are as follows:

*I will start tomorrow
*I don't have time
*I have no energy in the morning, or after work
*I'm too busy
*I'm too old/ young
*I am not motivated

Sound all too familiar? When writing this list, I identified individualistically with every single one of them. I would think that most people would agree that the excuses listed above have been recycled throughout their life at one point or perhaps many times when pursuing some form of change. This was certainly the case in my life. This is a recognizable self-defeating behavior usually caused by the fear of failure and of the unknown. The unknown being the fear of commitment, dedication, action, and discipline. The fear of failure, the results not being there, what other people will think of them for doing something new and challenging, how will other people judge or criticize them if they fail. This is where the lies we tell ourselves are created limiting our success within the possibility that is right in front of us.

In order to combat the excuses made, I had to take a very honest look at them and at myself. By doing that I was able to strip away the dishonesty of the excuse and then that exposed the truth of it. Seeing it for what it truly was. Unmasking the reason why I lied to myself in the assembly of excuses. By doing this, I uncovered a bridge between the way that words and the things I said to myself created a positive or negative momentum and that the momentum conjointly dictated the direction of the avenue in which excuses were created or were non-existent. The way we talk to ourselves creates or destroys the opportunity for excuses to be shaped. The link is compromise, it means to settle. When I would speak negatively to myself it would cause compromise in my thinking, feeling and emotions. Settling for less and then fabricating excuses to justify not making the necessary changes to improve. Opening the door for self-doubt and self-defeat. A negative reaction sparking an influx of negative energies.

When I chose positive reinforcement, speaking in a language of positivity to myself, I had absolutely nothing to compromise. A positive state of mind enables production through ingenuity and activity. Opening many doors of possibility. In doing so I had no reason to lie to myself in an attempt to justify a shortcoming because in the absence of fear, it did not exist. Sanctioning the ability to initiate an opportunity out of the unknown. A positive action that overflows with probability and outcome.

Looking back at the list of common excuses with this new introspection, we can uncover what these excuses truly mean.

*I will start tomorrow- This is probably one of the most used lies by people. By saying that we will start something tomorrow what we really mean is I'm too scared to start right now. As many of us know, tomorrow never comes, it becomes a perpetual Groundhog Day effect as we continue to stall ourselves from starting. This lie makes us feel like we will start, just not today. It's quite a comforting delusion that allows us to go about the present day without a commitment to the future.

*I don't have time- Actually, we do. In fact, we have lots of time. Unfortunately, all that time presents the freedom to make up more excuses and waste the time that we do have in our day, doing nothing. Saying that I don't have time means I don't want to prioritize and put some time aside to accomplish or achieve because I would rather spend hours on social media or watch a show. There are twenty-four hours in a day. Sixty minutes in each hour. Fourteen hundred and forty minutes in a day. On average people sleep eight hours so that would leave sixteen hours per day to be awake and functioning. Imagine the positive yield taking twenty minutes a day to exercise your mind and another twenty minutes to exercise your body out of that allotted time.

Cranking up feel good chemicals in your brain to help stabilize mood and emotional flow for the rest of the day.

*I have no energy in the morning, or after work- The voices in our minds are amazing at camouflaging our fears for mental and physical exhaustion. Therefore, many people end up hitting the snooze button in the morning instead of getting up early and taking action to start their day. Or end up on the couch after work and dishonestly negotiate with themselves, raising a convincing argument that there is no point to pursue activity because of fatigue and then most likely refer to "I will start tomorrow." What is truly being said here is that laziness may be a factor, but is not automatically the sole culprit, but our intimidation of the commitment to the action is as well. Look at the alarm we set as our life. Every single time we hit snooze we are cheating ourselves out of valuable lifetime and the millions of possible connections to opportunities within those moments. The same goes for the couch. Motion creates emotion. Movement creates energy. Energy fuels action. Action is change.

*I'm too busy- I hate to break people's hearts but when a person says they have been too busy regarding responding or paying attention to another person, what they unequivocally mean for the most part is that they have been busy living their own lives without the other person's presence and have not given much attention in regard to their feelings because they are not a priority. The same is true when people tell themselves they are too busy to start something new, make a change, or take action in their life. No one is ever too busy to make time for something they want. So, what is being said with this excuse is that we do not want to make the time because we fear the interruption of the convenience of our broken record like habits. Fear of change and the work involved. Fear that we will not get the result awarded if we try.

*I am too old- I am afraid of how hard it will be because I have convinced myself that my age permits success and people will make fun of me for making changes in my life when it's not a common time to do so in the judging eyes of society. This excuse can be flipped to "I'm too young". Positive change never has an expiration date until the day life physically ends. There is a never-ending affluence of available positive energy, so every single person is entitled to as much of it as they want. The more used, the more engineered. It is a reciprocal cycle. Age does not matter. Too young or too old are no longer viable excuses. The timetable of life is up to each and every person.

*I don't have any motivation- That's adorable. Perhaps if you did not have any food in your fridge your definition of motivation might change drastically. The motivation is always there, we sometimes need to find new incentives or inducements that will trigger our reformed inspiration. It's easier to talk ourselves out of motivating ourselves than to take the first step in a new direction, or so we commonly think. You, yourself are all the motivation needed. Once we can learn to believe in ourselves, inspirational influence is bountiful all around us. It just takes dedicated focus. Someone else's form of motivation may temporarily help but in-house centralized motivation is the key to success. You must build it. If you do not believe you are motivated, then you will not be motivated. If you choose to believe that there is motivation all around, you then you will see motivation every step of the way.

The enemy is distraction. Distraction comes in so many endless forms and is always readily available. Social media platforms are weapons of mass distraction. Boredom, laziness, procrastination, and self-doubt only exist when our fear distracts us from acting. The most common fears that people are afraid of that cause the need to search out distraction are the fear of failure, the fear of success, the fear of how you will look and the fear of losing.

I had to teach myself a new way. A new way to think and identify with the reasons I chose to lie to myself. Again, as I have mentioned previously, I had to understand the root of the issue first so that I could formulate my battle strategy to collapse the fraud in my thoughts which were disabling my ideas. Tracing my fears back to my childhood failures and looking at why they still affected my mind so many years later. Wreaking havoc on my will. The will to pursue what I wanted in my life. The will to find a way. The will to change what I needed to be to become happy. My trauma related issues from my impaired childhood development were at the forefront of reasons. The feelings I felt of rejection, ridicule or not fitting in after I was unable to understand things or be like everyone else, set off my defensive nature to protect my ego. Therefore, shutting down and not doing anything to improve my situation, experience, or environment. Telling myself why bother. I will just fail like I always do. This is where the excuses started for me. Excuses enable procrastination. Procrastination is the house that shelters insufficiency.

I feel that many people share the same patterns when lying to themselves, convincing themselves out of what they want to change or implement into their lives. Some will overcompensate by constantly talking about what they will do, posting it all over social media, but then do nothing except create excuses. Often blaming external factors as the source of their failure to do so. I believe we are taught by default throughout our lives by our family members, our friends and loved ones to stay inside our comfort zones. That Change is dangerous and scary. The unknown of the results can be disadvantageous to a lot of people because of the fear of failure and the judgements that may come with that. I found that in my depressed states throughout my life that I listened to everyone else except myself. That is probably why my depression had such periods of longevity. I knew I could be doing better things to make myself happier but chose to opt out instead. It wasn't until I adopted the same supportive nature for myself that I would exhibit it to other people I knew that were in the midst of the early first steps of making change in their lives. Why is it that we can be there for someone else but not for ourselves?

The fundamental sway in my ability to stop making excuses and start doing things to make improvements in every aspect of my life was as simple as this. I stopped listening to myself and started talking to myself. My way of thinking had been so wrong for so long. If I continued to listen to that I would never make any changes whatsoever. Making it obvious to me that if you do not believe you can do the task, you will avoid taking the first step to do it and make excuses. This creates failure in completing the task. Pedal to the metal on the feeling while pumping the brakes on thinking.

When I talked to myself and was encouraging and supportive while being assertive, that is when the magic happened immediately. Changing the belief in myself to one of self-efficacy. Believing that I could complete the task and I deserved that accomplishment in doing so. And with that satisfaction of accomplishment comes the momentum to move forward. Encouraging more belief in myself and my abilities. Thus, creating self-confidence. That confidence provided the framework for the reconstruction of my will. With will power and self-confidence together they make the recipe for courage pie. We all know that everybody likes a tasty piece of pie.

Of course, life has many obstacles and uphill climbs. Everyday has new sets of challenges that must be faced. Life gets busy and overwhelming. When I do find myself returning to past patterns of self-defeat and default to excuse making, there is a source of inspiration that I consistently lean upon when times get tough to help me pull through. It is a true classic literary masterpiece. Allow me to share it with you. It's a story of a little blue engine that is pulling a train full of necessities like food, toys, and candles over a mountain. She volunteered to do so after several other locomotives that were more powerful and experienced had declined for their own various personal reasons to not help after the original train carrying the goods broke down attempting to go up the mountainside. The little blue engine had never been over the mountain. Was not a powerful engine in comparison. The little engine was too small. Yet, she would go for it without hesitation or excuses. With the power of courage, positive reinforced thinking, self-confidence, and sheer determination of will, she believed in herself that she would get the task accomplished. "I think I can." "I think I can." "I think I can." She repeated to herself during the most difficult part of the upward climb until she reached the top of the mountain and then was able to deliver all the goodies to children in the village below. "I knew I could!" "I knew I could!" "I knew I could!" she happily rejoiced to herself. From the book The Little Engine That Could.

To break the pattern of habitual lying and constantly making excuses which lead to talking myself out of going after the changes that would greatly improve the quality of my life, I made this my daily mantra. "I think I can." Every small step in a positive and forward direction will change your life as you know it. For anyone else struggling with mental illness, or anyone having difficulty in their life in general, these small steps and shifts in thinking become monumental in momentum and value. Breaking the cycle of self-destructive behavior like self-doubt, self-defeat and replacing it with self-respect and self confidence that hails from self-discipline. Opening an entirely new life in a new world, every new day.

There is no easy path in the world of self-improvement. I want to be clear and honest about this. It can be uncomfortable and requires hard choices. Sacrifices. But there is reward in every new direction. Gratitude is a wonderful word but without action it is meaningless. You can write down all things you are grateful for every day, and it may spike your mood for a while, but let's be honest here, it won't make your bed for you. It is very easy to be grateful when things are good in life, when things are going our way. This is when it is easy to be positive. To feel blessed. To regurgitate all the overused cliches and catch phrases regarding self-love and positivity. Real change when it comes to self-destructive habits whether you do or don't have a mental illness does not matter when it comes to facing the hard truths about overcoming fear and making changes in your life. It's easy to abandon an action plan when things get tough. It's easier to give up than to go for it. Lies and excuses will always be there waiting for you with open arms. It takes dedication to the discipline of being honest with ourselves. Not just when it is convenient. Not just on social media. It was in the hardest moments that challenged me to not give up that taught me the most about myself. It was in the weakest moment of my life that I found out how strong I truly am. It was at the end of my lies that I found my truth.

The mind will consistently make excuses to keep you safe inside your comfort zone. Nothing amazing or life changing happens within your comfort zone.

If you think you can, you will.
If you think you can’t, you won't
Either way, you are right.
It's your choice.

CHAPTER 11

A SPOONFUL OF HONEY

In the war of ego, the loser always wins.
Buddha

My Ego had placed me on the top of the world. It led me to believe that I was invincible up there. Untouchable. Perhaps at one point, the only place left where my swollen head could fit comfortably somewhere. The world in which I stood upon was contrived of fraud and material things. Possessions and the identification with, attachments to, and the stories that come with all that. A number of years before I attempted to end my life, I was very successful in sales. I was surrounded by big ego personalities and adopted what I could learn from them all. The more successful I became in my career, the bigger my ego grew. I was very quickly propelled into management due to my charisma and being relentlessly result oriented in my pursuits. The higher I climbed in job status and earned more prestigious titles, the larger my ego grew. I was hired to bring results through my careful and militant perspectives on metrics and data conversion to opportunities in sales. I became very well known in the industry I was in and excelled extremely fast. I loved training and helping others become more successful as well. As time went on, I became selfengulfed, when unrecognized for my achievements I would become bitter. Sometimes angry. Oftentimes resentful and jealous. My lust for power and money took over and I lost sight of what made me successful which was compassion and eagerness to learn. My ego told me that I knew everything. That I was always right. It told me that I could not trust anyone who had a different opinion than me. In business it became my way, or the highway and I damaged many relationships by not caring how I got to obtain the best results possible. I became entitled. Bullying my competition. Everything that was good and prosperous was because of me in my egocentric point of view. It wasn't about the team anymore; it was about my team. How my team reflected my direction. Everything was about me. This would end up costing me my position. Not only once, but with three jobs in a row, over the course of six years. Delivering crushing punches to my ego. After being let go from my last job I was lost, devastated and angry. Suddenly all the things I stood upon as though they were sacred, began to crumble very quickly from underneath me. This perhaps contributed to my rapid downfall. My personal and business relationships were heavily taxed because of my ego and the blindness to my own arrogant and self-centered behavior. I blamed everyone else. Pointing the finger in every direction except towards myself. My ego would not allow me to see things for what they were. Instead, my ego told me that I was just fine. I was right. Everybody else was wrong. I had a very lavish lifestyle and loved to spend money. Unfortunately, my finances were drying up rapidly like a small puddle on a hot summer day as I continued to spend recklessly. I was always out and about, shopping, restaurants, lounges. I dressed like a movie star and was overly generous with what money I had left. My ego basked in the spotlight, being Captain Cool Guy. Buying, everyone drinks, shots, paying for bills, big tips on bills, showing off like I was a millionaire. Meanwhile, I had no food in my fridge at home and could not pay my bills. It became more important to look as though I was still financially successful than to face the reality that I was broke and getting buried alive in debt. My ego would not allow me to show the world that I was breaking down. My personal life was a disastrous mess. My self-centered actions were the reason I destroyed everything good that I had. I pushed the people who cared about me the most the furthest away. I became resentful towards them. My ego would remind me that I did not need anyone, but me. I had to start selling off all the possessions that I had left to survive. As I lost these material objects that I identified as a part of who I was, my ego compensated by cranking up the distortion of my perception of reality. Lying to myself that I would be fine. Overtime, I would lose everything. I was stripped bare. Leaving behind an empty shell. Nothing was left inside. My ego still would not allow me to ask for help. I was above that according to my ego. I was drinking daily to forget. I was back in theatrical form pretending to be something I wasn't. Lying to myself and anyone I came in contact with about how I was doing. I could not let anyone see the truth. I was too proud. All the while, a perfect storm of my life's failures, losses, heartbreaks and the shame and guilt that accompanied all that was forming in the skies behind me. About to unleash the wrath of the Shadow Monster upon me again. Like it had been waiting for this consummate moment to take shape. Its beady eyes smiled as it licked its chops, carefully remaining hidden in an attack-like position. I began insulting myself, telling myself that I was worthless, I had nothing to offer this world other than failure and hurting others. I hated myself. No one could ever love me. It was impossible. I was left alone with myself, I had holes throughout my identity where there used to be things that I no longer owned. I had no idea who I was. And right at that very moment, lightning flashed from the sky above, striking me down. The Shadow Monster attacked. Biting into me. I could feel its venom rushing through my veins and taking hold of my mind. Enter major depression. Exit all hope.

As I came into this world unconditioned and began growing from an infant to a small child, I did so with an instinctive and intuitive nature about being. Somehow, I had somewhat of an understanding of the world even before I could speak. The observation of the world around me was the language that I learned. My state of consciousness as an infant was one of pure awareness. As I grew into a small toddler, I learned how to play and use my imagination to create. Sensory. My mind had no filter or limit, and I was without a definition of my own identity. Everything in my being came organically to me. As more interaction and experiences within my life took place, I began to develop ego by being in an ego-centric state of mind. I suppose one could say that the world revolved around me in this state. Not possessing the ability to comprehend another person's perspective on a situation, only how it related to me. Childhood trauma causes wounds that are notably damaging during this egocentric period. This is when my Ego began to take over to protect me from my reality. Developing into a forcefield that would shield me from harm and commence the introductory formation of my identity. Sadly, like many other adults I had never evolved past this primitive egocentric state. Falsely identifying with my ego as what I thought my identity was. An identity that coped with confusion, disconnection, and the loss of love that I experienced. Compromising the understanding of values of achievement, relationships, and perspective. Learning to identify with the values even though they may not hail from positive origins to receive what I thought was being loved.

Ego is how one views themselves. An unconscious section of the mind that identifies with traits, beliefs, and habits. Becoming an inflexible identity that are the thought patterns, ideas, and beliefs of personality. Ego defends this line and will reject anything that attempts to cross over it that doesn't belong inside the box of confirmed thoughts and beliefs.

It was my ego that demanded that the world and all the people in it should be as exactly as I thought they should be. Winning and being the "best" became the most important priorities. Wasting so much precious time measuring up and marveling in my success based on how well I believed I stacked up against others. In the world of the ego, if you have more than other people then you feel better about yourself. Having more money makes you feel more privileged. Accumulating awards, accolades and titles were the complimentary counterparts that only added to the non-stop swelling of my ego. A continual flex.

It was at this level of ego consciousness where the problems existed and flourished. This is where my inner peace became virtually impossible, and success was bitterly unenjoyable because I was always striving to be some other place that I perceived to be better.

Taming all the wild radicals in my head like anger, hatred, despair, jealousy, fear, anxiety, and depression that all lived in the various parts of my ego. Dismantling the ever longing need to satisfy the call of my ego and the insistence to living up to an unattainable external standard. Outrunning my ego in order to tire it and slow it down. Discombobulating the anguish of not being able to fit in the common mold of conformity of an existential false world I had created with my ego. I became a minimalist with attachments, possessions, and people. Eventually letting things be of everything I feared to lose. Once I realized that stuff, things, people are not the core of my happiness the easier it became to let go. I also became a minimalist with my thoughts, emotions, and behaviors. Breaking many bad routines and self-destructive habits. In this world of consumerism which is pushing us to the brink of insanity with advertising, social media, celebrities, censorship, and the media dictating narratives, shows that it does not end painting a grand Illusion of all these incredible lives, people and the products needed to justify all of this in the mind as the only way to be happy.

Becoming deliberate with everything around you that it serves you. Not that you serve it. The newest cell phone, new car, new house, new whatever blah blah blah and the next new thing comes out. You are convinced by external sources that you have to get it in order to be happy, being led to make sure to post it so you can show it off your impeccable consumer instincts that make you stand out in a crowd, even though the crowd you stand out in is made up of people just like you.

Gaining understanding of the interrelation of the unhealthy ego allows you to open up to an entire new level where letting go of people becomes replaced with letting people be that are bad for us and serve no purpose other than maintaining negative energies like stress, worry and conflict. Ego holds onto every existential, lust, fury, control, accumulation of never-ending void filling things so you never have the opportunity to free your mind and become happy with yourself and what you have. Excess is the filler, the mighty distraction. Keep buying more things that are not needed and it will create happiness! Stockpile shoes that will never be worn, clothing that when bought gave a dopamine rush but now collects dust in the closet with the tags still hanging off them. Boxes full of gadgets, outdated technology, and toys, full of must have things that lost their trending novelty. The latest phone that doesn't do anything more than the last one that was released six months ago but is twice as expensive and comes in a new color that will certainly get mass approval and recognition from your brainwashed peers.

We attach ourselves to the things that make us look how we perceive other people want us to be. This does not create any happiness internally as it is all artificial, in fact it is detrimental as it divides who we are from ourselves. When I secured commandment of my ego, I was able to connect with who I was at the most basic level. Becoming one with the idea of me, not what the ideas of others looked like. I no longer searched for validation from anyone, especially strangers to help fill the void of the uncertainties of my insecurity. I shed the skin that was not comfortable to me because it was the facade of what I thought other people would like me better that way. Ego separates the mind from reality. It is a perpetual personal fantasy that is delusional based from fears of inferiority. Sometimes it's a battlefield where a big ego and a frail ego are at war within the person as it was with me.

Ego is a misguided sense of pride associated with feeling superior to others. The purpose of ego is to maximize social status on various platforms like power, wealth, education, and popularity. Arrogance is a dominant trait of ego. The driving force of Ego is self-interest. Invariably seeking out approval, validation, and accolades at any price to establish that you are always right. Ego is defensively rigorous and resistant to the difference of opinion, feedback, critique, and suggestion. Egocentric people like myself often will not care how their actions affect other people, replace kindness with judgement, think they are the best and everyone else should respect them, possess distorted perspectives of entitlement, and blame everyone and everything else for their failures because limits and defects cannot exist within the ego. This is the same for narcissistic personality disorder. The two are quite interrelated. Very difficult to see the differences as a big ego and narcissistic tendencies are overlapping in their definitions. The greatest difference in my opinion between them is that a narcissistic person sees only through a self-magnified lens. Creating a larger-than-life version of themselves that is unrealistic and has expectations of others that fall under this scope. A narcissist will have a very frail ego and will shatter if criticized. A narcissist will lie pathologically to obtain whatever it wants without remorse and use passive aggressive deceit to manipulate anyone it can. I certainly had crossovers of both. Many people with inflated egos are narcissistic. Every narcissist has an out-of-control ego.

Self-esteem is the evaluation of how much a person likes themselves, accepts who they are, and is comfortable within their own skin. Many people with low self-esteem will develop big egos to compensate for insecurity. I myself had tremendous confidence at times, pride in my achievements and a larger-than-life ego while having incredibly low self-esteem. In fact, huge egos are commonly a symptom of low self-esteem. Like myself, many people who feel very weak inside are constantly trying to prove to the rest of the world that they are more than they are, instead of proving it to themselves for the sake of their own contentment.

Confidence hails from one's own capability. It's a feeling that is being sure of oneself and capability without the need to flaunt it. Confidence is celebrated internally without being loud about it. It's not a superiority thing like ego. Many people feel confident within the constructs where capability is present and prevails. The lack of confidence comes from areas where capability is not as prominent, or as easily accessed.

For me and I would think for others, confidence helped me to get ahead. Whereas my ego and narcissistic traits held me back. Awareness is the sharpest point on the arrowhead, pinpointing the target. Through work, ego awareness is very possible and like anything else once you can accurately pinpoint the source. Study your own repetitive narratives of yourself inside the story of you exposing the external kicking and screaming behaviors of ego.

In our society we are taught to let other people validate our value and worth. We seek appreciation and individual recognition from those around us. Stemming from the abundance or lack of love or attention received from our parents as very young children. In essence this creates low self-esteem, weakening our own value we place on ourselves. Overcompensating with ego and narcissism. Social media is the perfect arena where people can pretend to be all the theatrical things, they are not but wish they could be in other people's eyes. I had been guilty of this myself. During the lows of my depression, I would post pictures in hopes of validation. It seems to me that society and social media are working together to dumb down the world. It is a narcissistic breeding nightmare. Emphasizing the connections on social media more so than connections between people in real life. With every second person pretending to be something they are not. Fabricating overvalues through lack of imagination chasing instant gratification through approval. Celebrities (many, but not all) are the biggest cause of misleading narratives and unattainable warped perceptions of what life is. What reality is. What beauty is. Their lack of responsibility and disregard for the impacts of influence on young minds is utterly disgusting and disturbing. What is even more saddening is that there are many truly profound individuals who are in the purest and most genuine form out there to help and influence every soul that they can without rewards like validation and likes. Ego is absent from their campaigns. The distance between confidence and ego are galaxies apart. Choosing a less arrogant path to relay their messages. Instead of trying to prove themselves to the world, they simply remain genuine and original to their purpose which isn't entirely about self-promotion. Natural beauty is a rare gem these days and that is what is wrong with social media and the world today. Flaws are beautiful. They make us different, unique, and memorable. The pressures of perfect beauty are destroying young minds at a catastrophic rate. Teen suicide is skyrocketing. Imagine how quickly this pressure could be relieved from these young impressionable minds if ego was replaced with confidence and healthy self-admiration. The need for egocentric validation would dissipate. Imagine if all the people that post about Mental Illness, did something about it instead. Now that would be truly so powerful. I bet it could move mountain ranges.

Here is a list of actions from my battle plan that I do every day no matter what to combat my toxic ego which allows my self-confidence to flourish:

- First Day Mentality- Approach everything you do like it is new and exciting. Like the first day. Be a student. Exercise the mind by reading, writing, learning something out of your comfort margins. People always say to live your life like it is your last day, I personally think this is the worst advice ever. If you knew it was your last day alive you would be in a chaotic state of panicked mixed emotions, twisted thoughts of regret and fear, attempting to fix and resolve so many things at once. That does not sound like a positive day of production to me. Instead, I choose to live as though it is my first day. Like a sponge absorbing everything I can and challenging my mind to embrace its energy and awe. Like a child would at the first visit to an amusement park or the ocean. Channeling the raw energy of humility by opening the mind to learn and understand genuinely in a state of wonderment.

- Moral Inventory- I consistently write out my good and bad thoughts, feelings, behaviors, and habits. Taking a few minutes every day and critique them in an encouraging manner. Weighing them on the scale of balance. This becomes the magnetic gauge of your moral compass.

- Transcend your thoughts forward- The ego wants us to stay attached to what was. I started to learn how to dictate the direction of my thoughts. Meaning I could project feeling and emotion into ideas in the future. Placing myself there by visualizing it happening. Manifestation. By doing that I was able to begin training my brain to think differently and take new actions towards where I wanted to be in my life. The past is over. Learn from it, forgive, and move forward. The present and future are excited for your presence. Ego does not thrive in the future.

- Positive Conversations with Myself- I had to drastically change my inner dialogue from very negative and pessimistic to positive and opportunistic. No more abusive self-destruction. The way we talk to ourselves reflects what we think of ourselves. How we talk about ourselves is the most important dominator in how we feel about ourselves. Daily personal affirmations/incantations stop toxic ego in its tracks. Good morning, Pep Talks with myself every morning always fires up the circuits! You can do it!

- Stop Complaining and Blaming others- When we do this it's your ego attempting to control your present thoughts and emotions negatively. Stop it right now. I complained because I wasn't getting what I wanted even though I did nothing to get it. Blaming is self-victimization and that in turn, is the host of your daily pity party. Redirect yourself for not doing everything you can to make your current situation better. Hold yourself accountable and then take the necessary action. Forgive others and yourself. Small steps add up to big changes quickly. If you catch yourself complaining, correct it immediately by asking yourself why in the world are you letting something get to you like that?

- Lose Expectation- Trade in your expectations for appreciation and your state of life changes instantaneously. Expectation is control driven by ego. Appreciation is acceptance with gratitude. Your ego can't relate to this and does not understand how to manipulate it. Think of expectations as the bars that hold together a prison cell. The less expectations, the less bars. No expectations of people or outcomes, no more bars. No more prison cells. You are free!

- Purpose- Following your purpose instead of passion. The alluring fires of passion can blow out just as fast as the spark that ignited them. Passion is very important and can lead to finding the path to one's purpose, but it's emotional and sporadic. Purpose is the reason why and is focused. Purpose is greater than you, therefore it is unselfish and giving. Not just about you. For example, my purpose is to help as many people as I can by sharing my experiences no matter the cost, in hopes that my words reach someone in the desperate moment of depression and help guide them home. My purpose is to inspire, to teach, to understand, to be strong for those who can't be. The voice for those who are too afraid to ask for help. That it is okay to be lost, hurt, or given up. That there is help and you are not alone. Passion is good. Purpose is great.

- Humility- Every day I wake up thankful for what I have no matter how good or bad things are. Smiling at the world. I shed materialistic fantasies for simplified reality. My pride is no longer allowed to conduct my personal affairs anymore. Ego and pride are best friends and can be very persuasive with negative peer pressure. You must break them up every single day for the rest of your life. I had to stop judging others based on my own shortcomings and the traits I did not like about myself.

- Standards- I created a new priority agenda that was set on this principle- this is good for my growth and happiness then do it. If it is not, say goodbye to it immediately and don't look back. This included habits, behaviors, people, and situations that were negative, toxic or growth stunting. I also created the standard of learning. Every day I immerse myself in learning more about myself and how that can benefit others. I also constantly improve my understanding of new and exciting topics and subjects by reading, studying, listening, writing, and sharing.

- Control- I always had to control everything. People, situations, outcomes, optics, image etc... I micromanaged my own micromanagements when it came to trying to control people to do what I wanted from them. It drove me to the brink of insanity at one point in my life as I felt the tight reigns of control loosening and eventually disappearing. I would overthink and analyze everything to the point of spinning myself out of control. The cycle would continue endlessly. My ego held people hostage through expectation. By letting what I could not control be and accepting that the outcome was not up to me was the most important lesson I learned. It brought me more peace and happiness.

- Focusing on helping others become more successful. The most important remedy for me by far out of these eleven steps. Paying attention to other people's needs, desires and goals allowed me to put aside myself absorbing ego and to focus on others. By doing so, I began to develop a sense of purpose and actualized a service within myself that was not about me but about helping others. Altruistic in my flow regarding all my relationships, not seeking approval, taking credit, recognition, or the spotlight because I was more concerned with what I could give to others in need. This step helped to lose the need to be somebody impressive and to concentrate on working on the way I could positively influence and impact others without seeking validation and reward.

- I simply stopped making everything about me. I slowly taught myself how to surrender the need to always be right and to prove others wrong. This in turn, aided the decomposition of my defensive mindset. Learning how to take a big deep breath before popping off when met with a difference of opinion, critique, or change. A more neutral attitude towards adversity. Replacing judgement and criticism with admiration and support. Doing what I could to offer input for accomplishment instead of looking for all that was wrong in someone else's plan or idea. Offering suggestive mitigation when I could, instead of harsh criticism. Learning everything I could from the experience as a whole. Fundamentally extracting the power from my ego and empowering a true state of humility and quiet confidence. Letting go of people and things is a form of control. Our ego never really let's go of a person and this usually turns into a conditional sentence where a grudge or judgements are put into place because they did not live up to our expectations. Letting people or things be as they are is true power. This empowers you and alleviates the weight of ego. Just let it be. You be you and let them be them.

If you find yourself feeling stuck in your life. Life doesn't feel right or good. If you feel disconnected or unhappy with where you are. You have difficulty making personal progress due to black and white thinking. You have a history of bouncing from one toxic relationship to another. Connecting with yourself or other people is challenging. If you feel like something is thoroughly missing in your life. You have an unhealthy relationship with yourself. If you are ready to heal and make changes in your life, perhaps some ego work is necessary like it surely was for me.

Releasing myself from attachments of my ego allowed a paradigm shift in how I viewed myself and others. Opening space in my mind for creativity, learning, forgiving, and letting things be. Detaching from expectations and judgements removed so much built-up toxicity in my mind. More vacant headspace for humility and grace. A healthy balanced ego can be a part of the working team that is me. Having a healthy sense of self admiration and self-confidence is like a big spoonful of honey. And just like my granny used to always say to me "a spoonful of honey will always get you further in life than a spoonful of vinegar."

CHAPTER 12

THE MONARCH BUTTERFLY EFFECT

"Don't be afraid. Change is such a beautiful thing", said the Butterfly. Sabrina Newby

It was a warm summer morning in early June 2002. The sun was beaming, and the sky was sea blue without a cloud. I was hunched over my very close friend's tombstone. I was hugging it so hard, and I did not want to ever let go. My body was convulsing with the hardest tears I can remember crying. My tears felt like punches to the gut from a heavyweight boxer. It was the first time I had visited him since he was killed only a couple weeks before. I was terrified to go that day; I knew I was going to break down hard. I felt so guilty, I felt like his death was my fault because I wasn't there to protect him, like I always had been. He had been murdered, shot several times in the head. I was in Edmonton at the time of his death. To this day I still wonder if I hadn't gone to Edmonton that week would he still be alive today? I lived just two blocks away from him and would accompany him daily on whatever he needed to do. He would call me even when he just wanted to go get a Slurpee and I would go with him. I suppose I was his muscle. He was half my size standing five foot six and weighing about one and twenty-five pounds but commanded ten times the respect that I did back then. I was a goon, an enforcer. He was "the Boss". There were far more dangerous, bigger, and tougher characters in our crew, but he and I had formed an incredible friendship and I guess that's why I was always with him. Although small in stature, his smile was bigger than anyone else's I have ever known. He was always laughing, always joking. He was very generous and kind, never rude or aggressive. I had spent some considerable years putting my time in with that crew. Running with the biggest and baddest men I had ever known. Into the wildlife. As I continued to hug him (his tombstone) in the graveyard that morning, I started to talk to him. Even though I knew the police had bugged his tombstone and had surveillance all over his grave site. I spoke to him for about an hour, telling him over and over that I was sorry, I was so sorry. I was ugly crying. I had so much pent-up anger and pain. I wanted to hurt someone so bad. My thoughts were twisting as the sky of my mind was cast over with violent thunder clouds swirling and funneling together about to create a very destructive force. At that very moment, a monarch butterfly gently landed on the top of his tombstone. Providing a very necessary distraction. A calm to the storm in my mind. It perched there and gently opened and closed its wings. Like it was waving at me. Like it was him acknowledging me. I have a tattoo of a butterfly on my back, and he always made fun of it saying, "look at mister big tough guy with his cute little butterfly." and burst out laughing. I could hear him saying that and I laughed out loud. It was the first time I had smiled in what felt like a century. At that very moment I knew he was speaking to me; it was his way of telling me that he wasn't mad at me or that I should not blame myself for not being there to save him. He had sent that butterfly at that exact moment because he knew I wanted to do something vengeful. I was so consumed by the Monarch Butterfly that I did not notice that an undercover police vehicle rolled up and the gang unit detectives inside were watching and filming me. When I did look up at them, they were waving at me and then they mocked me, like I was a big cry baby. High school bully mentality at its finest. It was a bit infuriating, but really it just made me realize what pathetic immature clowns they were. Being a highly publicized event, it had drawn a lot of media attention and the police wanted to make their presence known and they had a job to do.

The orange, black and white butterfly flew away as I stood up. I watched it dance its way through the air until it disappeared from my sight on the far corner of the graveyard. Walking over to my motorcycle, I could feel their judging eyes on me. I just smiled and blew a kiss at them and then rode off. I was pulled over about a block away from the graveyard by another undercover cop car. Two more gang unit detectives got out of the car. They asked me how my visit to his grave was and stated that it was sad what happened to him but then undermining said "that's what happens when you are in that lifestyle." I said thanks for the tip. I asked, "are we done here?" They turned around, got in their car, and drove off. A lot of things changed for me when he died. The importance of that day would serve as the initial beginnings of what would eventually become my metamorphosis many years later in my life.

Butterflies have many different meanings to so many different people from all walks of life. Often a very spiritual representation of many beautiful things in this life and in the afterlife. The Butterfly is a symbol of metamorphosis and unequivocal transformation. The analogy of this animal's development emphasizes the ability to move from one state, perspective, lifestyle to another in beautiful form. A symbol of new life. Leaving what life, it has known behind and courageously departing from the darkness of its chrysalis and finding its way to the flowers and gardens of a new life, illuminating all the way. The winds carried it to its purpose. The butterfly is regarded as a symbol of rebirth and self-discovery. In many cultures the butterfly is viewed as a visitor from beyond the grave of family and loved ones who have passed on. Showing up randomly and gracefully at times when we are saddened by loss to remind us that the ones, we love are connecting with us from the dead.

There are approximately eighteen thousand species of butterflies in the world and somewhere around one hundred and sixty thousand species of moths. One of my favorite butterfly species is the Monarch Butterfly. It is one of the most studied and iconic butterflies in the world. Monarch butterflies have bright orange wings which are laced with black lines and boarded with white dots. Famous for the seasonal migration millions of monarch butterflies migrate from Canada, south to Mexico for the winter. Monarch butterflies are native to North and Central America and spread to other warm places where their preferred food is milkweed. There are two species of monarch butterfly that are divided into two groups: the Western monarchs who breed west of the Rocky Mountains on the West Coast of North America and overwinter take up some sun tanning in Southern California. And the Eastern monarchs, who breed in the Great Plains of Canada and return to Mexico/Central America for the winter. The life cycle of the monarch butterfly is truly amazing. The female butterfly lays each cluster of eggs separately on a leaf of a milkweed plant, attaching it with a bit of natural glue-like liquid she secretes. A female should lay between 300 and 500 eggs for two weeks. After a few days the eggs hatch into larvae otherwise known as caterpillars. The caterpillar's main job is to grow so they spend most of their time eating. They will only eat milkweed, which is why the female lays eggs on milkweed leaves in the first place. Spring and summer Monarchs are in the egg stage for three to five days, caterpillars about ten to fourteen days, chrysalis form for ten to fourteen days as well, and an adult Monarch will live two to six weeks. Fall monarchs, meaning they were in the egg state in the middle to late summer, will live approximately six months. These fall monarchs will not reproduce right away as the spring/summer Monarchs did. Instead, they will instinctively fly south to Central Mexico which is a three-thousand-mile-long journey. Millions of Monarch butterflies will arrive every year at the same time between October thirty first and November third. Día de Muertos or the Day of the Dead celebration in Mexico is based upon this miraculous timing of this migration. Mexico has an intricate spiritual relationship with these Monarch Butterflies. Science suggests that these creatures are following a type of magnetism from the atmosphere, but Mexican folklore tells us that these butterflies are actually the souls of the deceased. Visiting Earth on these holy days to visit relatives to provide comfort. During the three-day celebration of The Day of the Dead many people will dress like Monarchs, decorate their altars with Monarchs to honor and remember their ancestors. A truly phenomenal and wondrous sight.

These Monarchs that made their way home to Mexico will be the first generation of the next year to fly north. It can take anywhere from four to six generations to make their way to their northernmost breeding grounds in southern Canada. The next time you see a Monarch butterfly in the upcoming spring, they are not the same Monarchs that flew south in the previous fall but if personified, this would be the great-great-great grandchild of the Monarchs that did.

The monarch's main source of self-defense is its colorful pattern that makes it easy to identify. The distinctive colors warn predators that they're foul-tasting and poisonous. The poison comes from their diet. Milkweed itself is toxic. The Monarch butterflies have evolved not only to tolerate but to use it to their advantage by storing the toxins in their bodies making themselves poisonous to predators such as birds. Here's where Monarch butterflies get crazy and absolutely blow my mind. As the days get shorter and the weather cooler, they know it's time to abandon their breeding grounds in the Northern United States and Canada and head south to the mountains of central Mexico where it's warmer. Some will migrate up to 3000 miles. Upon arrival, they huddle together on Oyamel Fir trees to wait out the winter. There are so many monarch butterflies in these trees that their sheer mass will often bend these gigantic trees over with their weight, because there are millions upon millions of Monarch butterflies taking refuge in the branches. So how is it possible for the monarchs to make such a long journey? Insects have super tiny brains. They use the sun to stay on course. It's like a navigational tool to them but they also have a magnetic compass to help them navigate on cloudy days. They possess a special gene for highly efficient muscles that gives them an advantage for long-distance flight. During the course of their migration these beautiful butterflies will face high winds, torrential downpours, thunder, and lightning storms, freezing cold nights, extreme heat, the destruction and deforestation of their natural habitats, pollution, and poisonous pesticides, and not to mention the cast of many different predators along the way. The Monarchs need to rest, drink water and feed on the nectar from a wide variety of flowers that produce sugars and other essential nutrients. In doing this like all species of butterflies, pollination occurs. Pollination helps the reproduction of healthy plant life. Butterflies prefer larger flower heads to perch on. The proboscis (long tubular tongue) and its legs collect pollen while they hunt for nectar. They feed/pollinate during the daytime when flower heads are as open as possible. Butterflies have spectacular color perception even better than humans and can also see ultraviolet light which makes flower markings very distinct to them. Butterflies cover far greater distances in their travel which ensures coverage of equal amounts of flowering plants in a larger area. While bees are known as the most proficient pollinators, butterflies hold their own in the world of pollination.

Imagine that small little beautiful butterfly, it's wings fully grown spread about the size of a coffee cup, that weighs less than a match can overcome all these incredible odds. Countless people don't know how to drive in their own city without getting lost or having to check with their phone or navigation system. Amazing to me is that these butterflies are relentless in their migration that is the perfect substantiated example of a purpose. They will not stop until they reach their destination, or they die doing so, to continue their unique life cycle. Regardless of how tired they are, they continue to fly,

Most people will never have a strong desire to get to their purpose in life, like the monarch butterfly does. The next time you think it's too tough, think of that beautiful orange, black and white polka dotted monarch butterfly. Because it is outworking you, it has better discipline than you. And only the instinctive belief that has it within itself succeeds in its purpose. If human beings could adopt the same principles with our brain power because we have more functional brains than butterflies, I think what we could achieve would be limitless. Most people are lazy. I don't think there's a day that a butterfly says to itself that it's not going to fly anymore. I'm going to wait till tomorrow to start flying. The next time you see a Monarch Butterfly, take some time to observe and admire this incredible animal, granting us the opportunity to imagine the hard work and discipline it takes that butterfly to achieve its purpose and the incredible metamorphosis it went through to become such a beautiful icon of transformation.

The significance of purpose in the Monarch Butterfly's story is that it signifies the truth about transformation. Without purpose there is no transformation. Without transformation there is no purpose. Purpose gives the direction in which to focus our energy and motion towards. Once purpose is discovered within us, that is when we will begin to transform our lives. When purpose takes over, I realized it was far greater than my sum. That is why I fought against having a purpose beyond a basic measure, because my life was always about me, and I was too scared to believe in myself and something bigger than I was. It took all my depression, anxiety, pain, anger, frustration, loneliness, bitterness, entitlement, jealousy, self-righteousness, and fears to combine into a perfect storm that took my life up in its funnel cloud spiraling me out of my control as thunder and lightning pummeled everything, I had thought had, misconstruing value into obliteration. Purpose as a noun by definition is something set up as an object or an end to be obtained. A subject under discussion or an action during its execution. For me, purpose in life means to remain agnostic to the route itself but ultimately devoted to a faith in a higher power other than ourselves. Creator, Creation, the Universe, Religious or Spiritual practices, whatever it is, it is completely up to the individual. The only requirement is belief. That belief will be the needle of your compass. Belief is the anchor to your purpose.

Once I was able to find my purpose, which in hindsight I had always known, that is when I began my transformation. I needed a way to create a template to help rewire my brain, to learn how to believe in myself and a higher power. The universe, energy, manifestation, and materialization of thought, giving out positive vibrations without an expectation of receiving anything in return, transcendence of mind, being able to project my future inside my mind and visualizing and feeling it so my brain could rewire this into its code becoming almost like a memory that had not happened yet.

I developed an easy system to help keep on track of my continuous growth throughout my metamorphosis. It's easy to manufacture obstacles which are emotional patterns of self-victimization, and suffering. We are programmed not to use our abilities and gifts to their fullest potential, instead we fill that emptiness with blame, anger, misdirection, resentment, fear, and our addictive nature of self-destructive behaviors. The Transformation Triad was created to combat these detrimental patterns. A model of interchanging expectation for appreciation through three key essential considerations that helped me to change instantaneously.

Imagine a triangle. A very common geometrical shape. The most common triangle is the equilateral, having three even lengths of sides with three congruent angles. For visual imagery this triangle will do, however during experiences the angles and sides will change, forming obtuse and isosceles triangles but the three essential points will always remain connected.

At the top focal point is Self-Discipline. The key to all transformation in ourselves and in our lives. Self-Discipline requires daily dedication, energy, and action. Through discipline I learned to stop the routine of bad habits, replacing them with positive daily changes that were healthy for me, mentally, emotionally, and physically. I learned how to hold myself accountable by being brutally honest with myself and not compromising my direction with any excuses. I stayed focused on goals, missions, and purpose by executing a daily growth plan through newly created routines to challenge my mind and body. Most importantly I finally began to keep going when I would normally give up because that was no longer an allowed option to do so.

At the bottom right side focal point of the triangle is Self-Respect. This is obtained through our self-disciplinary actions and provides individual standards and values within. I learned to accept both my weaknesses and strengths which lead to inner growth. I began to believe in myself and treat myself and others in a better manner. Through Self Respect eliminating sources of negativity such as environments, people and habitual behaviors become part of the daily routine. By recognizing patterns that were detrimental and replacing them with new character-building actions or activities, I was able to learn my true worth, what I stood for and what values I represented. This would provide the internal strength I required to reconstruct while experiencing setbacks and failures.

The bottom left focal point is Self-Love. Without first respecting ourselves, we cannot fully love ourselves. The standards of our Self Respect open new doors to Self-Love. For me, Self-Love was learning to reach a higher regard of self-sufficient happiness and well-being while simultaneously losing codependency of people, places, and things. No more negligence and dropping many things I had held on to so sacredly that did not belong to me anymore. I began to take care of my own needs and not settling for anything less than I deserved. Becoming understanding and compassionate towards ourselves changes our own internal conversations. This launched a constant state of positive energy and action with respect to me, inclusive of a recycling resource of true internal happiness.

Looking at the three essential points being Self Discipline, Self-Respect, and Self Love, it is paramount to understand the interactive relationship that all three points have with each other. That without the points connected the strength of the triangle disappears. Therefore, all three points must remain working together to maintain structure and balance forming a trinity. Transformation becomes established once the mass between the insides of the triangle is identified as Belief. It is belief in these three points that hold the triangle together and produce the constant flowing energies travelling in both directions from one point to another. Self-Discipline creates Self Respect which in turn creates Self Love. This trio creates belief. Belief is the anchor that holds it all together. What this allows is the triangle to change shape during different experiences, meaning the length of the sides and the angles may change in correlation to which point is in immediate challenge. The strength of the triangle being believed allows this flex and to maintain its form. Life will provide many opportunities in which you will have to rely heavily on Self Discipline and secondarily Self Respect leaving Self Love stretched further away from these points, but the connection and function of all three remains. People will interrupt our state of happiness and impeach our character, thus forming a triangle with Self Love and Self Respect as the closer two angles and Self Discipline stretched out forming a new shape of triangle. All three points glued by belief make these equilateral, acute, obtuse, scalene, isosceles, and right triangles an adaptable and consequential belief system template for ever evolving transformation and growth based on the individual's own reciprocity of energy within their personally designed construct. This became a moderated obsession for me and completely changed my life. The triangle can change its form many times a day and this is its power for our transformation. Once we begin our transformations with small actions and movements, we begin to grow. Continuous growth requires continuous transformation. Our thoughts, emotions, behaviors, habits, environments, perspectives, perceptions, actions, reactions, attitudes, energies, and our direction are transformable constantly and through the use of the Triangle of Transformation template that I created for myself, I was able to laser focus my energy into the most optimal outcomes. This became the origin of the assembly of my purpose. Transformation and purpose are nothing but words without each other's results and actions connected. Together, after a period of the darkest of darkness, purpose and transformation would form my wings, just like that of the Monarch Butterfly, after it leaves its dark chrysalis. Enabling flight to fulfill contribution to the world and to sustain life for others without any expectation other than contagious action that will help others navigate as they fly confidently into the unknown. Every person is a butterfly in the garden of life. Love is the pollen on each flower. Share that pollen with every other flower possible as you fly through the world exploring new and unknown gardens. Showcasing that transformation is the most beautiful purpose in life.

The butterfly effect is a chaos theory where a phenomenon from a miniscule change in a complex system can yield massive effects somewhere else. A dramatic representation of saying that the flap of a butterfly's wings in one part of the world could have profound effects on the weather on the other side of the world. Like creating a tornado or a typhoon. It does not mean that the butterfly itself provides the energy to create these storms, but the flapping of its wings represents a small turbulence within the atmosphere that causes a chain of events heading up a much larger chain of events many thousands of kilometers away. The small amount of energy from the butterfly's wings is the tiny change in trajectory that as it builds momentum travelling it gains more energy eventually altering the events within the system. This was introduced to the world in 1963 by Edward Lorenz, a mathematician and meteorologist who invented chaos theory regarding a new formula in predicting weather systems.

So how does the butterfly effect play a role in our lives? The model from chaos theory teaches us that a small change within a complex system has dramatic effects causing an enormous change in that system through a series of chain reactions. Just like the Monarch butterfly is a small part of the larger scale system of mother nature, our ideas and actions as people are a part of the extraordinary system that is our world. I believe that a small idea put to action can change the world as we know it in the most colossal way. Effecting the construct of the system to change through many chain reactions. I believe that we all can change the bigger systems with small actions that will reach people across the world that in turn will continue to prove the theory's hypothesis is correct. Need proof? You are reading it right now.

CHAPTER 13

THE OSCAR GOES TO...

I think the saddest people always try their hardest to make people happy because they know what it's like to feel absolutely worthless and they don't want anyone else to feel like that.
Robin Williams

Robin Williams was my favorite actor and standup comedian growing up and still is to this day. From his rise to stardom in the TV series Mork and Mindy all the way to his most current projects that included many diverse roles and wild characters. Some of my outright favorite movies of his are The Fisher King, Awakenings, Good Will Hunting, Patch Adams, Dead Poets Society and The World According to Garp. Of course, there are so many other incredible movies that could easily be added to this list.

In my opinion Robin Williams was the best underrated actor in his time. He made every single role he took on so believable and relatable. I was very drawn into his performances. I often forgot that he was acting because of how powerful his emotional delivery was within the vast array of the characters he played.

In 2004, I had the honor of being Robin Williams personal security when he visited a bar here in Winnipeg. I was a doorman at this establishment. I was asked to shadow him and make sure that nothing out of the ordinary happened to him. To basically ensure a safe environment and remove anyone that may compromise that. A few other actors and staff from the movie were present as well. The movie was titled "The Big White" which was shot over a few months at various locations in Winnipeg and surrounding areas. During that time Robin was very kind and generous with people throughout the city wherever he went.

When I was introduced to Robin, I had an abundant amount of excited energy built up and I kept saying to myself over and over in my head "Jay, be cool, don't ask him a bunch of dumb questions and tell him how amazing he is." When Robin shook my hand all of that went out the window and I could not contain my excitement and told him how I was his biggest fan and started asking him questions about various roles in his films. So much for my big plan to be captain cool guy. I explained to him why each of the characters he played made me feel such a range of emotions. That I felt connected to them, to him. He graciously listened to me and even did some on the spot impersonations of the characters I had expressed my fondness in. As soon as he was done chatting with me, there was a change, a shift, he immediately became withdrawn and instantaneously lost all expression on his face. His outgoing body language reversed. I'll never be able to forget his eyes. He was staring blankly at nothing and when I looked into his eyes all I could see, and feel was emptiness. Almost lifeless, yet still a small sparkle of child-like kindness. I have witnessed the life drain out of someone's eyes before and that is an awful experience but that is what his eyes reminded me of. In fact, they were the saddest eyes I had ever seen, but I recognized them from many of his characters in his movies. Particularly his characters in The Fisher King and Good Will Hunting.

However, as the evening carried on, whenever someone would come over to talk to him, he would impetuously snap back into character and compassionately play an outgoing Robin Williams, to not let anyone down when meeting him. He courteously took photos with many fans with tremendous energy and as soon as they walked away, he went right back to what I observed and interrupted to be in a depressive state. Almost catatonic. I found it heartbreaking and challenging to watch. I had to wonder if Robin Williams was acting in his movies or was, he acting in real life. Something that I could instantly attach to and empathize with. It was truly a defining moment in my life that night protecting my all-time favorite actor. We often forget that the famous people we idolize are actual people just like you or I, that think and feel the exact same way as us.

Sadly, years later, Robin Williams committed suicide by hanging himself at the age 63, in 2014. This came as a huge shock to the world. As most of the public had the conception of him to be always happy, joyfully upbeat, and always funny.

The hard lesson that I learned from Robin Williams's experience is that severe depression is legitimately an equal opportunity Mental Illness. That no matter the level of intelligence, talent, passion, brilliance, wealth, fame, and power are not enough to protect anyone from the effects of depression. At some point no matter how big the distractions are in our lives; we all inevitably end up alone with ourselves at some time. The distorted perceptions of self will always resurface with Mental Illness. Over time those perceptions can become more significant than actual reality. Left untreated in extreme cases, leads to suicide.

I shared a very similar distorted view of myself and my place in a world that offered little promise of happiness or hope. I could be surrounded by people that admired me, but I always felt alone. As though I did not belong. I suppose I have always felt like an outcast, an outsider in my own life. As a way of compensating for these feelings, I often turned to humor as my way to cope. I have always had a talent for spontaneous comedy and have had little fear of making fun of myself to get people around me laughing. It was a connection to them that provided an instant bonding gratification for me. A quick fix to fill a bottomless pit. I wanted everyone to notice me, to like me and at some times to fear me. Depending on which of the million different people I was at that moment.

I had become an actor in my own life. At times I was unsure of when I was genuinely myself or if I was acting in a characterized version of myself. A lot of overlapping between the two. I was an imposter in my own life. It started for me when I was a young child. In a span of a few years dealing with the tumultuous relationship of my parents leading to their separation and divorce, moving households many times, enduring what seemed like a custody battle that had no end in which at times I felt like I was a weapon, blaming myself for their parting of ways, starting over at multiple new schools, being sexually abused by multiple people, bullying, physical abuse from a principle and others, the emotional, mental and physical torture I endured had left me feeling destroyed. Ripped apart. Stripped of my right of happiness. My innocence was stolen with the caress of my cheek. I was broken into shattered desperate pieces. I felt like I had been scattered all over all the wrong places to just get blown away in the cold wind. Leaving me with the feeling that I belonged nowhere. Having to reinvent myself so many times as a little boy, I became a chameleon. I learned how to change my skin out of discomfort to blend in. I wanted to be seen and unseen at the same time. Camouflaging my true colors that I was sorrowfully color blind to. Crying out for attention to be noticed for being different while hiding behind the truth. The truth being that I was never comfortable in my own skin. Please notice me, but don't notice me for who I am. I hope you like me because I'm trying to look the same as everyone else. It's terrifying being different as a kid. I was always trying to fit in anywhere and everywhere else that I could. Perhaps this is what caused my suspended durations of loneliness and depression throughout my life. Never knowing who I was, only who I was trying to be. Creating what seemed like millions of versions of myself constantly. Invariably due to the many changes in settings as a child, this carried with me deep into my adult life.

At a very young age I learned how to act tough and angry when I was scared through assimilation. My transitional environments were very temperamental. Sometimes, I would hurt myself when I got upset. I hit myself a lot, punching my own face and head as hard as I could, I cut myself on occasion too. It did not matter how many times I shed my skin, I still hated being me. I could not outgrow what had been done to me. I could not outrun the monster that was beginning to surface in the dark shadows deep inside my nightmares that still were awakened in my mind. I was a silly happy go lucky boy at times. I was also full of hate and pain. I despised how I felt being so unbalanced all the time. Like my blood was cursed with something potent correlative to Blue Coral Snake venom. Living and dying a thousand times a day. I hated the people that hurt me, but I wanted them to like me or love at the same time. A very conflicted and contaminated soul I was.

My life has always felt like I was being improvisational in a predetermined screenplay that I have played the lead actor in. As I have regularly attempted to spontaneously create or recreate my ever-changing character to the scripts that seemed like my life had been pre-written for me. Almost like I was a stand in during my own life's dress rehearsal. I was playing the part of life instead of living my life. Acting through the motions, without feeling the appropriately connected genuine emotions. Years of projecting myself into a fantasy world to escape reality as a child, regulated the catalyst for this behavior. Losing myself often within the assortment of the collection of various cast members I had become. All of them shared one common theme, trying to be someone else in hopes that people would like me. That I could fit in. I became the standup chameleon. I have always been wild and untamed. Radical and extemporaneous. Over time the merge between who I was and who I was trying to be became seamless. Indistinguishable. At times this would propel me into being the class clown, the life of the party which I embraced with open arms as I loved to make people happy and laugh. Soaking up all the attention. Other times, the standup chameleon was outshined and hid cowardly in the background. Enviously observing everyone whilst internalizing how to mimic what I ascertained as their strengths. My envy of other people that seemed to be happy with themselves developed into resentment, jealousy, and anger. Inspiriting a villainous side of me to arise. Criminal. Vengeful. This was the Segway to my metamorphosis into a monomaniacal madman motivated by lust and fury as an adult. Constantly in search of attention from women in hopes of regaining what I perceived not to receive as a child. Being sexually abused by a young woman in my early childhood was the icing on the cake. My sister and I were still living in the same house. I was five, going on six years old. The babysitter we had looked after us would put my sister to bed early and then she would tell me that we were going to play a secret magical game that I was not allowed to ever tell anyone about. She was seventeen. She would kiss me, take all her and mine clothes off and then tell me to kiss her all over her naked body. Then she would put me inside of her. I remember the sound of her excited breathing climaxing. I got to have ice cream afterwards every time. This went on for months, every time she came over to babysit my sister and I. Being raped by a woman at such a young age directly affected my conflicting opinions on trust as I grew up. I was too young to formulate proper ways to work through the damage that this did to me. Hypersexualized behavior at a very young age that would continue with me predominantly throughout my years. Misinterpreting lust for love sent me down a never-ending unfulfilling pursuit, with only temporary gratification that left me feeling more alone afterwards. I was in a state of despair and even when I had the love of a woman it was never enough to stop me from sabotaging the relationship when they got too close to me. All I ever wanted was someone to love me but as soon as that happened my internal armed guard went into attack mode finding a way to start a war. I broke many hearts in the misguided pursuit of preserving the condition of my empty heart, never entering a state of love and trust. My anger became consuming. Hate began to fill the void left behind in my heart. Throughout my lifetime it was like I was split into two very distinct and different complexions of character. One was a scared little boy that wanted everyone to like him, insecure, lost and endlessly searching for love and belonging. The other was an angry boy who wanted people to fear him, tempestuous, violent, and felt animosity towards those who misunderstood him and hostility to the unfair life that he was imprisoned in. Inside each of those two characters existed a boundless constellation that harbored a million more variant roles that came and went in reaction to the circumstances of the wild ride of my life.

It was like playing a game of chess without fully understanding how to play chess. The pieces were all there and I could identify each of them, however I lacked the knowledge of how to manipulate them to advance or defend my position properly. The chess board was the experience of my life. The pieces on the board were the components of my interchangeable personality. Without a comprehensive strategy, chess is a losing battle. Every move becomes based on reaction. Much the same as my life and ability to remain comfortable within my own skin. Very difficult to heal that which you cannot feel.

A wild goose chase is an unsuccessful search for someone or something and ends up being a total waste of time because what was being searched for does not exist or is impossible to find. This would be a very fitting description of how I felt trying to find myself within the person I was a stranger to. The stranger inside of me was configured by the innumerable versions that had lived and died in the hopeless endeavor of finding myself. I was always looking to discover myself in other people, trying to find out who I was in everybody else, but me. I became well versed in making it look like I had it all together on the outside. That's what I thought was important to other people. I lied to them and to myself, so much that I believed it. When lies become truths, reality and fantasy are separated by a very thin delicate borderline. Feeling like an unstable blindfolded tightrope walk between sanity and insanity while high up in the wind, wearing cumbersome shoes. Later in my life, I would realize that trying to find myself in the created version of what I believed of what people would like me to be, was utterly impossible and in actuality, insane. Increasing the distance between where I was and who I was. Only adding more venom to the toxicity of the relationship with my depression and my other Mental Illnesses. My ego would develop narcissistic patterns in allowance of my insecurities that hailed from not ever knowing who I was. This is one of the clear dangers of Mental Illness. Lacking a true sense of self is like a dying hollowed out tree still attempting to house and shelter animals from the callous elements that are killing it.

Incessant reinvention of myself to fit surroundings when I was not understood or felt uncomfortable while being dictated by the unresolved issues from my younger years, presented the birth of the chameleon. The actor that could change in and out of characters to adapt to the environment in which I was in. When I was young I did not like the idea of it, because it felt out of my control. Unbalanced. Reactive. When we are kids, our lives, environments are dictated for us. Sometimes at us.

It is in those defining moments of experience when we are young that shape our ego, identity, and self. I remained stuck there, mentally, and emotionally kidnapped for most of my life without any growth. It was not until I was able to dichotomize and articulate these experiences and accept what happened to me back then was wrong and not my fault, but was a rite of passage, a footing, an anchoring point that I could build strength and courage from. The root of growth. I began to change the navigation of my thoughts and I became able to see where I had been blinded from for so many years, my vision quickly evolved into seeing everything as an opportunity to learn more about myself. Shedding the self-victimization which had enslaved me in fear. This led to rapid growth. With that growth came a positive perspective on a restored way to chart my redirection. I also realized that I had formed an alliance with the negative thoughts from my past. Allowing them to wreak havoc in my present-day relationship with myself, and that would also have a trickle effect on others in my life. By holding myself hostage in situations that happened so long ago I kept myself in a state of immobilization. Trapped by my fear of letting it be of what happened and embracing the unknown of becoming who I was. Inside the awakening moment of letting myself be from my fear of people not liking me and belonging anywhere else besides to myself, I immediately went from attempting to blend in as a chameleon to showcasing my brightest colors and my boldest patterns changing as many times as I could in a day. Being as many versions of myself as I possibly could. Not only embracing change, but I also created it. In fact, I could change the entire setting of my environment so that it fits me because it is all in my mind. We are not meant to be the same person every day. That is truly absurd. Biology is always perpetually on the move. It can be ruthless and beautiful harmoniously. Life is in an always changing state. Diverse. Progressive. Adaptation and evolution are the instigating and influential forces of change in nature that ensure its continued success. I had to ask myself, for someone who loves and studies biology like I do, why would I not follow this natural course of action?

The inconsistency of not having a stabilized environment growing up subjected me to a nomadic lifestyle both physically and mentally. Always wandering lost in my thoughts of where I belonged. Living with parents, then from parent to parent, grandparents, home to home, place to place, going from school to school and the constant shift within all those settings had an unambiguous impact on the level of comfort I had within my own skin. The moment I began to feel comfortable enough to begin to grow somewhere, my entire world as I knew it was uprooted and taken away from me only to be relocated and replanted somewhere else. I tried to act like the other trees that had been growing in the comfort of the same soil and surroundings since their beginnings but every time I was dug up and replanted, it stunted my growth. Searching for my place in the new environment. As many of the other trees around me were beginning to blossom, grow and reach out for the sky, I was still the same small size. Often hidden in the shadow of their growth. I wanted to be the biggest tree there was so I could have huge branches full of leaves that were a haven for so many species of animals. To provide shade from the hot sun and a place to call home. I wanted to be seen from far away. That did not happen. Instead, I felt small, insignificant, inferior, overshadowed, and overlooked.

I know that many people, just like myself, are many versions of themselves as well. Some are good and some are bad. Oscillating between them. Many of us wear disguises as different actors within our own lives. It is through the harsh scales of comparison and judgement that are pushed upon us from an early age that begin this transformation within us. Most often our parents, through their actions, reactions, and the way their attention or lack of, is communicated to us as kids, shapes the mold of our inner conformity in hopes that we will please and be like what someone else wants us to be, so that we can be admired. Sought after praise when we accomplish something. When that is not met, that is when the actor inside us takes center stage. For some, it's an easy and controllable substitute in character. For others like myself, who were trapped in an everlasting state of loneliness, it becomes second nature. Putting on the show in hopes that someone will like it and that will lead to them liking you.

As I have made my way through so many scenes in this movie called life and got to the place I am now, I have come to understand a few things about all of it. All these characters inside me, are me. They all come from the circumstances of my experiences. It is within the construct of our perspective that dictates the perception of these versions of ourselves, whether we need to pretend to be something we are not, to fill the emptied and drained parts of us left by those who did not grant us the attention, care or love we so desired. Some of us will go too far and morosely not find our way back to ourselves. This was the story of my life without question. Nevertheless, all those millions of people I had experienced from beginning to end, shaped the embodiment of who I am. Once I took on the mission to be able to identify with and understand this, I was able to accept this as an opportunity to reconnect with myself. To find out who I truly am by honoring who I was and who I had been. It also allowed me to trace back to all the roots of the controversies within my incidents that caused me to become a chameleon or actor and redefine them in a way that I could learn more about myself by studying what caused me to not be myself in these circumstances. This became a newfound freedom as I glued all the million pieces of me together. Intrinsically creating the chameleon that was now comfortable changing its colors in its own skin. No person is the same as they were the day before, even though the Groundhog Day effect might make us feel otherwise, we are in a constant state of change. It is up to the individual to find that beautiful merge of identity that balances the chaos and art of the characters inside their mind. Life itself is a stage meant for many performances. Just take a few moments to yourself every day and appreciate the miracles of nature that are playing out before your very eyes. The theater of miracles

Every so often in life when all seems lost, the perfect moment arises to find ourselves

CHAPTER 14

SCAR TISSUE

When you realize that there's a name and a description for this condition that you thought was insanity, you've identified the problem, and now you can do something about it.
Anthony Kiedis, Scar Tissue

Sadness and heartbreak felt like suicide. Anger felt like murder. Distance felt like abandonment. Happiness felt odd and foreign. Falling in love seemed to be impossible and felt like being a continuous inconvenience. Loving someone felt like losing all control. Losing someone felt like dying. Feeling normal felt like emptiness or nothing at all.

Everything felt so unstable. Confusing and unclear. A wavering sense of who I was. My self-image frequently changed just as quickly as my rollercoaster of emotions. I was extremely sensitive, like that of an exposed nerve ending. The smallest things could trigger explosive volcanic-like reactions from within my core. Once I exploded there was no way in sight of calming down. The volatility of my unpredictable emotional state led to turmoil in my relationships by acting out recklessly and impulsively. At times very selfishly.

It is impossible to think rationally when caught up in the drowning undertow of overwhelming riptides of emotions. Making it strenuous to find your bearings or to stay grounded. When faced with these emotions I would say hurtful things, act out in dangerous or inappropriate ways in turn making myself feel more guilt and ashamed of myself afterwards. It was a painful reciprocating cycle that showed no promise of escape. The dysfunctional patterns of thinking, feeling, and behaving I was exhibiting were a result of lifelong habits that I needed to change to free myself from the grips of the monster in the shadows. I often felt so empty inside. Depleted. My emotions would shift in such extremes within the same timetable of an experience. Anger, sadness, and anxiety would expose themselves jumbled and muddled together like mud in the eye of my emotional storm. I was in a constant state of panic from fearing that the people I cared about would abandon me or leave me for someone else. Even though when they pulled me close, I would push them away. I would best describe most of my romantic relationships as very intense but equally unstable and not always long lived. The way I felt about people in my life would dramatically change in a heartbeat from one moment to the next and I did not understand why. In the fog of my insecurity, I would abruptly lash out or make impulsive gestures to keep the other person close to me. A backhanded sense of control. I would recurrently do things that were dangerous or unhealthy like driving recklessly, binge drinking, using drugs, getting in fights, indulging in illegal activities, going on spending sprees, and anything else I could get myself in trouble with. I was unable to untangle myself from the mess of these reactor distress coping behaviors.

It was difficult to wrap my head around everything. Tempestuous skies within my mind were clouded with turbulent and swirling thoughts that I could not control. My unrestrainable behaviors were the result of this, and they were killing me. It felt like everything in my world was ending. It was like my house was on fire and all I could do was just sit there watching everything slowly burn down around me. Why was I like this?

I learned from the scars left behind from my own experiences that people do not necessarily have toxic relationships with other people, but more likely they have a toxic relationship with themselves. That was unquestionably the case for me and most of my relationships. My inner toxicity attracted the same person with a different face and name repeatedly. I invited that and allowed it to happen, looking back at it, but we rarely see it that way when we are in that moment. As well, my own toxicity made it impossible to execute proper self-reliant choices. Crying out for dependency to all the wrong people, places, and things. I was stuck in the endless pursuit of the next woman who inevitably would turn out to be bad for my health. Ignoring my gut feelings about them and believing that somehow this time would be different. I had not set of true standards for myself which made it impossible to operate properly with another person. I did not even like myself, know myself or trust myself and that attracted complementary toxic people into my life. My toxic trait of searching for someone to rescue me from myself, to love me and make me feel as though the emptiness inside me would be gone, while fixing all the broken pieces of me and providing the life that was missing in the void of my own life, was a very unrealistic fantasy that I would continue to pursue to the brink of my own insanity without end. When I did have a good and healthy relationship, I sabotaged it and pushed that person away from me. Making sure that they never go too close. I did not believe that I deserved them deep down and always thought that they would leave me anyways. But when they left me, I hated them for leaving. It was comparable to being an air traffic controller giving out mixed communications to incoming flights and wondering why they all crashed and burned, while others either avoided the mayhem completely, or became so confused that they became upset while attempting to solve the mystery of the mixed messages and just flew away. Do not get me wrong here, there are people who are narcissistic psychopaths that destroy good people. Take advantage of others and do not care how their actions affect the other person. But if that pattern continues to be repeated in your relationships, then there is the question of your own toxicity towards yourself that needs to be addressed.

Admitting and accepting to being a toxic person is a hard pill to swallow for most people in the beginning of self-realization. It assuredly was for me. Taking a spoon of your own medicine can leave a very bitter taste in your mouth. My ego did not like it one bit. It is always easier to blame the other person in the relationship and self-victimize than to take responsibility for the choices made to stay with that person even after our guts have told us many times that we should not be with them. Blaming the other person for their inadequacies like lack of attention, admiration or dedication is common practice and makes it easier to feel sorry for ourselves and play the victim. This stems from our convictions of control and expectation. These patterns can also be the Segway to justifying cheating, having affairs and other deceitful behaviors while staying in the comforts of a relationship. I have been on both sides of that coin. My fear of being alone or abandoned resulted in staying with people who were toxic or becoming the toxic one myself in the relationship. It would appear to me that in a toxic relationship, the person who seemingly cares the least in the relationship often controls and dictates the trajectory of the relationship for the most part. It wasn't until I discovered through the process of my self-actualization that I had abandoned myself long ago in my childhood somewhere hidden in the scar tissue left behind from trauma. Running away from myself as fast and as far away as I could was the only way to escape the pain of distrust and betrayal. I would have to travel back to the times in my mind when I was sexually abused and confront the fears that were the result of those traumatic experiences. I would need to search through the feelings of the emotions tied to those memories and find a way to separate the betrayal and trust. Confront the years in my childhood that I felt abandoned and neglected, looked over or unnoticed during my parent's separation and divorce. By examining the associated measures of the impact of toxicity in the environments of those experiences that I would push myself to relive in order to gain a better understanding and perspective. I needed to learn how to trust myself and other people. The scope of introspection was targeted on my own brain, and I was about to become a sharpshooter.

There are trust and distrust receptacle areas in the brain. Two separate functions taking place in two different parts of the brain. Distrust is signaled through the amygdala and trust is signaled through the prefrontal cortex. Taking place in the prefrontal areas of the brain, trust is formed while the brain is assessing the predictability, credibility, and the nature of intentions of someone's behavior. Taking place simultaneously, distrust happens in the lower brain as we are assessing the level of threat that someone is projecting to us. In this same region of the brain is where the fear of loss is generated. Uncertainty is created in the mind when these two functions overlap. This created emotional threats to my mind and would invoke a state of fear. Once we have had a bad experience and begin to become distrustful of a person generally, that impression or imprint becomes deeply embedded in our brain and can be very difficult to dislodge the longer it is allowed to exist. I had to systematically learn how to hit the pause and rewind buttons to review exactly what happened. Otherwise, I found myself in a similar and familiar destructive pattern which was ongoing throughout my lifetime of carrying the weight of my pain and lack of trust dumping it on one relationship to the next. Never taking the time to look at what I could have gained in understanding from the experience while I was in the relationship.

Once I was able to reconstruct the old worn-out wiring of distrust into a newly formed stronger cable of trust, it was then that a cocktail of my brain's natural feel-good chemicals like oxytocin, dopamine and serotonin began to flourish. Learning to trust again created and generated new bonds that helped change the neurochemistry in my brain and trigger a new network of neuron activity. By implementing my concept of the triangle of transformation into this equation, I relied heavily upon the self-respect angle here to aid in eliminating toxic people from my current thoughts and emotions. Letting them be where they belong, which was somewhere else. Self-discipline would support this by keeping in line my daily actions to eradicate unhealthy habits regarding relationships. Stopping me from repeating the same detrimental patterns of my past. Self-love would play a role here as well reminding me that I did not need to let go of people as that was a form of my ego holding on to the reigns of control, instead just letting things be which for me was so much more emotionally disencumbering and freeing, as this took away any of the weight associated with it. When we are in a state of fear the conversations, we have with ourselves, and others are shaped by the neurochemistry of fear. Therefore, we become defensive and only think about protecting ourselves. The remedy to the brain's fear state are trust, empathy, and support. When someone shows concern for us or we have concern for ourselves, our brain chemistry makes a shift. We become calmer and regain composure and this allows us to begin to think in a constructive and productive fashion. When the chemistry in the brain switches from trust to distrust we often end up feeling betrayed. Fear in conflict changes our neurochemistry and also changes our persona. Once we make our minds up about someone, we too often set up to prove we are right.

We are conditionally addicted to being right. Always in attempts of validating our assumptions.

Taking an honest look at my life, really inspecting it truthfully, zeroing in on the facts not the feelings was the first step in self-discovery. Outlining the results of the facts of my experiences allowed the breakdown of how my habits and behaviors either benefited my growth or disabled it. By writing it all down it became apparent what I needed to do to change the non-beneficial habits into beneficial actions that served my purpose of self-improvement. Exposing the patterns of self-disrespectful behavior in which I could now better understand and introduce counterintelligence to combat these detrimental habits that wreaked havoc in my mind and in my life. I could make the necessary tweaks and adjustments with my newfound self-reliance as I grew the relationship, I had with myself. Sighting former dysfunction as an opportunity for supplementary function.

I had to learn that the nature of my mental illnesses caused impulsive behaviors essentially as a chemical complication in the management systems of my brain. Accepting that and as well, that I often acted before thinking about the consequences. It was important to recognize that these impulsive behaviors served a purpose instead of a problem. They were coping mechanisms for dealing with despondency. Regaining control of my behavior started with learning how to tolerate dejection and despair. Acquiring the new ability to tolerate distress helped me to press pause when I had the urge to act out. Instead of reacting to difficult emotions with self-destructive behaviors as I previously had, I learned how to ride them out while remaining in control of the experience. In childhood we all develop coping mechanisms. Coping mechanisms are the strategies that help to navigate through stress and trauma, manage our difficult emotions and adapt to overcome adversity. Adjusting our personalities in an attempt to maintain emotional well-being while faced with hardship of life's experiences. Balancing an emotional equilibrium with a positive self-image in the appearance of negative junctures in our realities while making the necessary adjustments to do so in the perceived arena of stressors. Commonly, negative life changing events and the negative variables that are its components are the bedrock of negative psychological stress. This stress associated with change comes from the brain having to adjust and adapt. Experiencing too many changes within a brief time period can overwhelm the brain, especially in childhood. Exposing my young developing mind to the feelings of not being able to control any of the things happening to me. I believe that this misguided perception at such a young age is the contributing factor in my low self-esteem, ADHD, depression, and the development of a plethora of mental illnesses or disorders in myself and many people alike. It would make sense to me that these coping mechanisms override normal brain function causing confusion and catastrophe chemically in the brain which results in an imbalance. The unusual demands of coping require greater energy and effort from the brain and perhaps this is what causes learning or cognitive difficulties and behavioral disorders in the young shaping minds of children facing emotional anguish though negative changes. The prolonged immobilization of the mind in its early developmental stages while being bombarded with elevated levels of stress from the accumulation of the onslaught of many traumatic changes could be the culprit to the retrogression of mental and emotional progress in my case.

These are the ways in which we adapt some attributes of our personality. Of whom we are. If you had a parent that was not loving enough or did not seem to pay attention, you may have made an adaptation to acting out to feel noticed or appreciated. If you had a parent that was angry, violent, or an alcoholic you might have developed a coping mechanism like becoming a comedian to evade their anger. Or perhaps you bottle everything up and become under spoken. Coping mechanisms developed in childhood are meant to be functional and flexible creating resilience for us early in life. But as the decades go on, they begin to confine our personality because we should no longer require their services. Alternatively, they become like an old beat-up suit of armor that we inconveniently clank and crash around in. I had to take an inventory of all the masks and armor that I was still wearing from my childhood as some of the pieces of the personality puzzle that were well past their expiration date. These age-old coping mechanisms serve as damaging retrogressive habits now. We should live freely and autonomously while no longer requiring these protections or defensive coping habits. Mental illness can cause these coping habits to present themselves every day. Habits can be difficult and exhausting to break, especially when they have been in place for decades. For me, the way to successfully remove these rigid habits was to replace them with fresh flexible adaptations and fluidity in actions taken to form new habits that served my purpose, not my past. This was only possible by again identifying the origin of experience that caused the behavior which would ultimately become a habit. Dissecting the thoughts and emotions that designed the change or adaptation in personality. With that information in the tool belt, I was able to begin building new habits because I had freed myself from the scarring feelings of the past experiences. Self-discipline and grit were the power tools I relied on to get the job done.

There is an appealingly insightful moment in life when all the broken pieces of who you were and what you have gone through all begin to take shape, forming and fitting together, revealing who you are now. When the realization hits you that all the traumas, tragedies, sickness, pain, and heartbreaks that you endured have created the strength of the character you possess now. That the tears were the release of pain that you needed to go through to continue to grow through. When a smile lights up your face when you can see how all the intricate pieces of the ever-changing puzzle that have come together to make an inspiring piece of artwork. Something to be genuinely appreciated and celebrated. The ugliest truths about ourselves can become the most fascinating and magnificent characteristics of who we are through self-examination leading to the path of self-actualization. Becoming fulfilled by finding meaning and being at peace with the scars left behind from the battles of the past. When we can learn to trust ourselves wholeheartedly because of our transparent intent in our actions is when all the doors open up for self-respect and self-admiration in its most authentic and genuine way. Unlocking the freedom from the need to follow the opinions of anyone else in our lives and be in a pursuit of possibility, instead of a pursuit of problems. Learning to accept ourselves through accountability helps to alleviate the toxicity in the environments in our lives. Self-respect is the superpower that protects all the progress made through self-exploration. Depression has less of a fighting chance when many of the preceding triggering determinants are removed. I learned this the hard way and that turned out to be the best way.
It truly is such an empowering and honorable moment when we can look upon all our scars and smile because we appreciate that we have earned the right to acknowledge them as what has made us unique and breathtaking.

CHAPTER 15

NO PAIN, NO GAIN

Pain will leave once it is done teaching you.
Unknown

What is pain?
What causes pain?
Why do I feel pain?
How long will pain last?
How is all emotional pain related to ego?
Can I change the repetitive cycle of pain with a new belief system?
How do I turn pain into a valuable lesson?
How is pain the best motivation for growth?

As I sat on the floor of an empty gym, I looked around at all the weights, the heavy bags, and all the various equipment and thought to myself how therapeutic it was to be there. No matter what mood I was in when I entered the gym, by the time I was done with my workout, I had released emotional pain through physical pain. I have spent the majority of my adult life pushing my body to its limits in many different kinds of exercise. Boxing, Traditional Martial Arts, MMA and Muay Thai Kickboxing, Military Calisthenics, Running, Pilates, Weight

Training, Cross Training, HIIT, Powerlifting. Each of these I have pushed through the presented limits of pain to get better, faster, or stronger. To gain new ground or territory I had to face the pain and smash through it. In weight training which I have dedicated my life to, I have made considerable growth through years of destroying the physical breaking points of my body. How? I realized that everything physical is actually mental. All limitations are created in the mind. Instinctive and manufactured fears combined with neurological messages sent to the muscles in my body. In bodybuilding the catch phrase "no pain, no gain" is a reference to pushing past the physical limits of pain while lifting weights to create growth in the muscles by making them stronger. The only way to accomplish this is by adding more weight to what is being lifted or by doing more repetitions in a workout which stimulates growth through repairing the muscles of the body afterwards. That breakthrough is rewarding mentally, emotionally, and physically.

Pain. Often is described as agony, discomfort, suffering, hurt, aching, torment, or misery. There are a few types of physical pain felt in the body caused by injury, sickness, or emotional trauma. Pain can be generalized or localized depending on what type of pain it is. The scale of pain can start from mild discomfort and slide all the way to excruciatingly debilitating.

Psychological, emotional, and mental pain can be described similarly as physical pain, but the difference is that it does not always originate from a physical source, although sickness, disease and disorders can be the route of emotional pain.

Emotional and mental pain commonly is caused by the results of situations such as other people's actions or reactions, trauma, loss, rejection, heartbreak.

The feeling of physical pain comes from our nerves reacting to injury or sickness and sending a signal to the brain. It's a form of communication to warn the body of the injury to further prevent more damage or to become aware of the sickness. The thalamus inside if the brain sends out the information to all the different parts of the brain. The brain then collectively processes the information and sends the message to the site of the pain.

It would seem that there are neurological similarities with physical and emotional pain and can-do damage to the other. An overlap of neurological responses. When I was in a constant state of emotional suffering, my body was in a state of distress as well. I was mentally, emotionally, and physically fatigued. A synchronically intertwined spiral of mind and body aches followed suit.

I found that there are two distinct types of pain. Both are characteristic to physical and mental. The first is pain that hurts and the second is pain that alters. Pain that hurts can be adapted to, mended, and healed usually within a moderate time frame. Pain that alters cuts deep and scars, removes part of us, changing our lives. This altering pain can overtime begin to mend and heal but it will require hard work and more pain to do so. The two have significantly different timelines and damage levels but share an analogous outcome which is growth. No pain, no gain.

For many years of my life, I held on to what hurt me. Sometimes consciously and other times subconsciously. I let that pain dictate my behavior in many ways. After decades of unsuccessfully attempting to bury the memories of the abuse and trauma from my childhood and teen years through my adult life, I in doing so created the hardwiring and imprinting in my brain of a dreadful habit. Hiding from the memory or the experience does not take away the scars left behind from the damage done. Instead, what this ongoing behavior taught my brain was to shut down when a new opportunity presented itself. Especially when it comes to relationships, love, and trust. I would shut off feelings to stay safe. There is an anonymous quote that says, "if you don't heal from what hurt you, you will bleed on those who did not cut you." This could not have been more accurate about my personal relationships. The brain's main occupation is to keep us alive and safe. It is within our state of mind that the feelings of memories can flirt with the lingering pain of the past, safekeeping them in the present moment's choices to protect us from experiencing the pain of the past even though the circumstances or situations are ultimately on a different chronological timeline. By attaching pain to a memory and habitually re-enforcing it through reliving it, it becomes a pattern that is hardwired in the brain. That is how a standard behavior comes to life.

Initially, emotional pain causes people to build walls that protect. To guard themselves. When I was hurt by someone, I immediately constructed a giant impenetrable fortress all around me. A monstrosity of an impervious structure. Equipped with large moats surrounding my fortress of solitude that were full of blood thirsty piranhas, high voltage electric eels and hungry crocodiles. Making it beyond the bounds of possibility that that same person could ever get close to me and hurt me again. Of course, this is all metaphorical, but in reality, what I was doing was overreacting to a present moment of pain by basing it on the data stored in the hardwired pattern of thoughts from my past ordeals. Meaning that instead of acting on the source of pain, be it from another person as the example, and then properly diagnosing the current symptom of the pain and how to analyze and overcome it. I would do the opposite and react to the source of pain, incorrectly diagnosing the pain because I was basing it on the past which resulted in being defeated by it, without overcoming it. Like a default setting. Doing the same thing over and over which only added more lifetime to the pain of my past. Roadblocking the healing process that I so desperately required. It is entirely up to the individual how long pain lasts. Pain runs its course, but our ego will emphasize the pain to remind us not to change. The ego wants to stay the same. Whether or not that is a good or bad state, the ego does not care. It wants to remain perfect in its controlled habitat in the mind. The relationship between pain and the ego is all about control. The ego will make us question how someone could not love us, or how could they possibly move on in their lives without us. Holding us captive inside the pain of that feeling. Centering all thought on an outcome that cannot be controlled. We sit and wallow in our misery extending the lifetime of our pain. The bigger the ego, the bigger the hurt when our sense of self is threatened, challenging our idea of our worth. I felt so much pain throughout my time because my ego would not allow me to move forward and learn how to heal in a healthy way. Depression clouds our vision of the present moment, crippling the opportunity of letting the past be so that we can live freely and productively in the current experience of the juncture we are in. Depression is all about the past. Anxiety is all about the future. Both share the common trait of the fear of the lack of control of either situation. Both depression and anxiety disorders stem from a situation in the past where control was unattainable while suffering an injury or tragedy causing pain. This is expressed in our behaviors. In our actions and reactions. When suffering pain, I would remain in a reactive state of mind. This mental state is endangered, and this results in compromised thinking that disables healing. The never-ending cycle of allowing this reaction to happen every time I was in an emotional conflict increased the amount of pain, enhancing the augmentation of more pain. The more pain I felt, the more I hurt myself by self-destructing and sabotaging anything good in my life that would have aided in my healing. Living in a state of weakened potential as my ego would keep me fixated on the unjustness of the source of pain and the relationship with that. Just like any injury, if we do not take care of it properly, it does not heal, and can get infected. The infection or sickness that comes from our emotional wounds when not healed is mental illness. There are not any band aids available for these wounds. It can start early in childhood. As an example, a young child can not measure up to the standard of their parent, the expectation of the child's physical appearance is a common reference point by that parent. Comments, insults, and actions regarding this by the parent cut into the child's self-esteem. As life goes on that child begins to develop a complex about how they look. The wound does not heal as they age and it gets infected with a mental illness such an eating disorder, broken mirror disorder or body dysmorphia. Constantly in a poor state of mental health as they are always looking for that perfect version of what they perceive it should be, even though they are looking into a broken mirror making it inconceivable and insurmountable to them. The pain that comes with that leads that person to never being able to feel good about themselves, no matter how hard they try. The unhealthy fixation of body image takes over and anorexia nervosa, bulimia nervosa, binge eating, anorexia athletica or related other disorders begin to creep into that person's life. The illness often makes them blind to what their body looks like, and the results can be horrifying and in extreme cases lethal. I developed muscle dysmorphia which is a body dysmorphic disorder that no matter how much muscle I built I always felt skinny, like when I was younger. I became obsessed with building bigger muscles to the point that I was taking so many steroids, eating eight times a day, and working out for two hours every single day. The bigger I grew, the smaller I felt. Which drove me mad. Insane. The years of being made fun of for being so small and skinny when I was young created a wound that allowed this sickness to infect my mind. The bullying that made me feel so helpless played its part in the pain that stimulated this obsession. My muscular body was a shield. It was intimidation. What it truly was is a protective suit of armor to keep everyone away from the scared little skinny boy trapped inside. I recall one time I had returned home from being away for a while and met up with a couple good friends for coffee on a patio. As we were catching up, one of them made a comment to me that I looked smaller than the last time they had seen me. I pretended to laugh it off but, in my head, it was like someone had just stabbed me in the heart a thousand times. My ego and mental health disorder went off like a fire alarm. I literally disappeared for two months, not showing my face in public other than the gym where I would work out for hours every day. I injected multiple types of anabolic and androgenic steroids and ate strictly high protein and fat-based meals seven or eight times a day. I returned to meet my friends once I had gained twenty pound of solid lean muscle wearing a t-shirt that would fit a small child so that it would be so tight that every striation in my muscles could be seen through it. We joke about it now, but that is the severity of that disorder. No matter how big I got, it was never big enough. It took many years for me to negate this way of thinking. I still am challenged with it in my present day. I'm always in the gym pushing myself in a healthy way now.

It took the dire severity of becoming so depressed that I wanted to end all the pain of my life by committing suicide, to open the eyes of my mind and learn how to see again. I have had so many amazing moments and experiences throughout my life, but depression blinded me from this. Just like anything, we become what we think about. As I concentrated the spotlight of thought on pain, that is all I felt. Producing a downhill domino effect on any good memories and happy thoughts I once had, knocking them down one after the other until they all had been flattened. When I was at my sickest point with my depression, I believed that a painful ending was better than endless pain. I believed this because I had lived my life circulating as the victim of the circumstances that caused pain to be the center of my inward attention.

When I made the decision to learn about all the experiences in my life and how they constructed me as a person instead of how they deconstructed me as a person, was when I was able to dedicate my efforts primarily on what caused me the most pain. I needed to be able to comprehend what caused it, how it happened, why it happened, when and where on my timeline of my life, and who was involved? So that I could catalog the exact results with the same questions regarding the impact on my present-day life. This would be my guide in distinguishing a roadmap of all the many paths leading back to the origins of my pain and then highlighting the way back to a newfound understanding which was liberating and empowering, opening my mind to see things in a new way. This was not an easy process by any means. I had hidden behind my anger from my pain all my life. Pain was the hub of my habits and behaviors. Repetitive meditations, countless documentations of my feelings and thoughts when reverting to victimizing myself when upset, celebrating forgiveness, removing expectations of control from the circumstances of the past, maintaining a growth plan that tracked my success in development as I made my way through the battlefield in my mind. Self-disciplinary action plans taught me how to embrace pain as an instrument of growth. I basically broke everything down about the incident into the tiniest fragments of the cause and effect so I could compartmentalize them before restructuring them into useful building blocks. Strictly analytical in the approach but not overthinking it. Simplifying the emotional aspect by removing blame and guilt from the experience to expose the injury/trauma/sickness for what it is. I relived the experiences and the pain that I had been harboring for decades. As I wrote down the compositional elements and the explanations on paper it was such an amazing emotional release. Many pieces of paper were adorned with tear drops. Big happy teardrops as I began to mentally, emotionally, and physically free myself from the prison cell of my past. Like the feeling of warm sunlight touching your face. The more I faced the pain, the more I began to understand the positive equity of the experience that caused it originally. Causation holsters a previously unseen value when the mind is opened up in a state of awareness. Awareness is knowledge. Knowledge is the facts of the experience and the ideas that come from that. This creates the connection to wisdom, which is how to apply that knowledge in the bigger scheme of your life with deeper meaning. Insight is the clear perception of life, knowledge, and wisdom. True understanding of the intricacies of your own life and the big, beautiful universe that your life is gracefully intertwined with. My newfound knowledge of the experience would reveal the fundamental elements that bore the harsh reality of the circumstances involved. I saw it as though it was in point form, a collection of circumstantial data. Determining the who, what, where, what and how corresponding with the trauma that was the nucleus. Putting that knowledge on paper,

I was able to study the information like a doctor would with a wound. How did the wound happen? What caused the wound? Why did it happen? Who was involved? Where and when did it occur? Was there an infection from the wound and if so where had it spread to? Wisdom would now take over once I was done diagnosing. Taking all that very useful data and using it to gauge rehabilitation and recovery. A healing processes. Reviewing my notes would illustrate patterns of behavior, habits. In order to heal I had to break those habits that were causing the pain in my life. Just like a doctor would create a treatment plan for the wound. Does the wound require stitches, how to treat the infection, and the various stages of aftercare? My newfangled insight of the overall occurrence taught me how to unchain myself from it. To stop routinely punishing myself with guilt and shame. Forgiving those who hurt me and wounded me causing pain and suffering. Understanding that the universe had made me stronger through these wounds by healing and repairing the core of who I am. That the experiences were trials of my character and that when I changed my perspective from victimization to victory, I was flooded with elation and exhilaration. Releasing me from the cage of pain while simultaneously inciting growth from that pain. The question was not that some of the things that happened to me were atrocious and wrong. The real question that my insight asked was how long I would continue to punish myself in a life sentence inside the unlocked penitentiary of pain I imprisoned myself in. The answer was never again. No more. Finally freeing myself to feel the wind, as I ran wild. A wild animal with a purpose, I had become. That purpose was to free as many others as I could from the cages that held them prisoner.

Some of the most fascinating people have been anguished from their pain which sparked their artistic brilliance. Musicians are a perfect example of this. So many songs are written by artists amid their pain that when listened to, we feel that emotion and we relate to it. It evokes personal feelings and stimulates our own creativity. Maybe we dance to the song, or write a poem based on the shared connection of pain, perhaps experiencing that music becomes a deciding factor in someone's life and they learn music to express themselves and to deal with their pain.

Without pain there is no growth. Without pain there is no creativity. I believe that a lot of the pain we feel is because we live contradictory to our own nature. By limiting ourselves from what we truly want in our lives. Self-inflicted pain does nothing good. Am I immune to pain? Not at all, I still feel pain often. Pain is necessary. Pain is the best educator in life-providing lessons. By transforming my pain into positive transitional outcomes, I was able to stop myself from transmitting my pain on to others. Celebrate the influential factor that pain often is the originator of the victories of change.

Through concentrated self-exploration, the more pain I embarked upon from my past allowed embracement through releasing it. Letting it be. Embracement means to accept willingly. To unconditionally understand. The more tears I shed, the lighter I became. Yet, stronger. A true feeling of freedom. I was transforming. The darkness of the chrysalis around me was getting lighter. I stretched out myself pushing through it and exposed my magnificent wings to the world. The imprisonment of fear, pain and darkness was over. When I finally learnt what pain had taught me, is when I learned how to fly.

CHAPTER 16

THE CEREBRAL SAMURAI

Think lightly of yourself and deeply of the world.
Miyamoto Musashi

The master control center is the brain and your nervous system. A power plant that produces processing power that controls how we react to everything. A synergetic network of neurons and fibers that turn data to action. Neurons send signals throughout the nervous system. There are one hundred billion neurons inside the brain. Every single moment, cells carry electrical charges which are impulses that transport messages throughout the whole nervous system. This allows it to make sense of the world while adapting to the conditions of our environment.

When we want to improve the capability of our bodies, we do exercises, we challenge our muscular and respiratory systems. While pushing our bodies through some form of fitness training, we elevate our brains chemically which in turn gives us a very positive feeling of accomplishment.

Many people follow strict workout regimens and chart the growth of muscle, the loss of fat, the duration or distance gained and are elated when the results of their hard work pay off.

We push our bodies in the form of exercise to combat aging, overcome weight issues, improve the way our body looks and feels, conquer insecurities, raise personal esteem or for overall benefits of improved health.

As someone who has dedicated so much to training my body and pushing myself to my physical limits, I began to ask the question, what would happen if I applied these same techniques in training my brain? Would the results be the same or perhaps even better? Could I establish a workout program for my brain and mind to grow stronger together with the intention to limit the symptoms of mental illness or boost a poor state of mental health? With the ambition to learn how to manage the state of my mind so that I could use the feelings associated with triggering depression, anxiety, OCD, ADHD to work with me instead of against me. Establishing a new balance into my brain, life, and mental health.

Your brain is not a muscle but acts like one in some ways. I immersed myself in learning everything I could about how the brain works biochemically and neurologically, how brain cells develop and how to make my brain stronger. After all, it is said that a healthy mind and healthy body go together hand in hand.

I was fascinated to learn more every free moment I had about how my brain and mind work. I read about neurology, cognitive psychology, and related brain sciences. I listened to leading neurologists, psychologists, and studied every related subject so I could understand it and make sense of it all. Then cross referenced all the data and information over and over. I began to understand patterns, behaviors, how environments affect how our brain functions either in a positive or negative way. How different states of emotion created altered brain chemicals to work or stop. That it is possible to continually strengthen your brain power and generate the production of new brain cells. It's like lightning striking throughout your brain as you experience new thoughts and feelings. New vibrations and electricity.

The distinction between the physical organ of the brain and the cognitive ability of the mind are that the brain is a malleable set of neurons that are ever evolving whereas the mind is a computer like learning machine that is perpetually adapting to its ever-changing environment.

The mind is always in a state of being a work in progress. Exposing new stimulation and exercises allows the mind to grow stronger, faster and become more efficient every day. Developing the mind daily by problem solving, overcoming challenges, strategizing plans, and accomplishing them, learning, reading and for me most importantly writing. These become like exercises for the mind and brain. When we exercise, we become healthier and more fit. The same goes for our brain and mind. Our overall mental health is improved from physical exercise as well as mental exercises.

The mind uses the brain, and the brain answers to the mind. The mind also changes the brain. The brain changes with every experience we have. Every second of every day. Meaning, that when people choose their actions that is done so in the mind as their brain will not do that because the brain merely responds to these unique experiences. The mind is responsible for how we think, feel, and choose accordingly. The brain inside our skulls is an extraordinary neuroplastic responder. What this means is that every time we stimulate our brain with our mind, it will respond with genetic, neurochemical, and electromagnetic adaptations. Growing and changing the structures inside our brain while building and wiring new physical thoughts. Neuroplasticity is the brain's ability to form new neural connections while adapting throughout our life. We are growing new brain cells all the time as well as repairing and restructuring the cells that we already have.

Understanding that the mind and brain are separate put me in the captain's chair. I could carefully acknowledge and choose what I built into my brain and how I wanted to change what was already built in by managing my thoughts and actions. With this concept, I would set up an exercise program for my brain and my mind. Brain fitness and mental self-defense. These exercises would develop into a cerebral workout that immensely improved the state of my cognitive, mental, and physical health in a symbiotic alliance of synchronic synergy. A fancy way of saying they all worked together to make me smarter, stronger, and more balanced. I theorized that if I could improve the functioning of my brain through stimulation and exercise that it would help regulate chemical balances which would then aid in maintaining a controllable level of mood and emotion. This would enhance the state of my mental health and reduce the symptoms of my mental illnesses. Enhancing the relationship between the states of my physical health and mental health simultaneously would prove this true. Let's get down to the nitty gritty of how to become a cerebral samurai.

Physical exercise is the first element of cerebral samurai training and the most important due to its multi-purpose applications. When we exercise, not only is it good for our body health, but it is great for our brain and mind health as well. As we exercise physically, it immediately causes dopamine, norepinephrine, and serotonin levels to blast off. Endorphins that are also powerful feel-good chemicals are released into the mix as well. This instantaneously encourages all kinds of positive adjustments in the brain like neural growth and development, boosts concentration, memory, mood, attention, focus, reduces inflammation, relieves stress, improves cognitive ability, which all together promotes a state of well-being. A power-packed medicinal formula to combat mental health challenges all in the form of physical activity. I personally believe that physical activity is particularly important every day. I like to go to the gym four or five times a week, go for bike rides weather permitting, daily walks year-round, yoga and various other forms of activity whenever possible. That seems like a lot for most people but that is what works for me. Dedicating just twenty minutes a day to physical activity will work for anyone and produce positive results. By enhancing the level of physical fitness, it will enhance the level of cognitive fitness. The more active we are physically, the more active we are cognitively and mentally. New muscles make new proteins that aid in brain cell growth. Stimulated in the quads, glutes, hamstrings, and calves. Another reason not to skip leg day. Go do your squats.

The second element of cerebral samurai training is brain fitness. Training the brain to be more powerful and effective so that it can adequately rewire what is already hardwired in the habitual programming of the brain while creating new connections between brain cells and brain areas. Sounds fun, I know. All we must do to achieve this is learn new things. New habits create more connections.

The newer things we learn, the newer brain cell activity there is. Integrating stimulating activities like learning a new skill set or incorporating new hobbies, learning a new language, reading new books, problem solving games like puzzles, crosswords, and chess, working with numbers. Basically, anything to get the brain to consider variable solutions to a new challenge will present great engaging exercises for developing brain fitness. Perpetual learning equals uninterrupted growth in the brain also known as neurogenesis. For me, writing, reading, constantly educating myself with new subjects, new hobbies, dedicating time daily to these brain exercises had a vital influence in the new and improved functioning and performance of my thinking cap. What was once a "loose screw" was tightened. Devoting just twenty minutes per day will promote a healthy and fit brain.

The "use it or lose it" principle applies here.

Mental self-defense is the third element of becoming a cerebral samurai. The progressive chemical and cognitive behavior that improves notably with physical exercise and brain fitness needs to be protected from the intrusion of dangerous and harmful antagonistic adversaries that threaten the state of our mental health. Those adversaries are our thoughts and learning how to defend against them is the way of the warrior in mental self-defense. Bushido which means "the way of the warrior" is the code of seven virtues that the samurai lived by. Adapting these seven virtues towards my thoughts invented a new robust mindset that was ready to defend and always protect.

*Integrity- When it comes to making decisions, integral thoughts are based on moral principles. Proper decisions.

*Courage- The courage to always do the right thing and not to give in to fear based thoughts. To fight the good fight internally, regardless of how others judge. To stand up to the bully.

*Benevolence- Balance the mind and thoughts with inner charity by having mercy and sympathy with letting thoughts be that require no defense. Why waste energy on something that does not require any.

*Respect- Respect everything because everything is everything. When thoughts are aligned, our decisions are based on self-respect.

*Honesty- Always being honest with ourselves and our thoughts.

This is the way to be able to change how we feel about our thoughts in a respectful manner to ourselves and others. Inner trustworthiness.

*Honor- Thoughts that are honorable, command disciplined actions that are true. Honor the experiences as lessons. This is the way.

*Loyalty- Remaining loyal to the values of what benefits our mental health. Safeguarding the relationship within, no matter what the external circumstance.

Practicing mental self-defense takes repetition. Repetition develops technique. Technique creates speed. Speed generates power. To get better at something, we must practice it over and over. As we practice doing the same thing or idea in repetition it helps build our technique. Once the desired technique is mastered then we can begin to do it faster. As the speed of the delivery of that technique increases, so too, does the power and effectiveness of it in its execution. Meditation helped me to slow down my thoughts and command them appropriately within the code of the seven virtues. Meditation for me, took on many different modes of practice. I did practice traditional methods of meditation where I would concentrate on my breathing, slowing everything down and carefully selecting my thoughts until there was silence inside my head. Somedays this would last ten minutes, other days it would last for hours. Meditation also came to materialize when I was out in nature, riding my bicycle or going for a long drive outside the city. Sitting beside a waterfall was an irresistible invitation to meditate. Once I was able to conduct the flow of my thoughts and trust my feelings about them, that was when I could begin to speed up my technique and become more authoritative with its delivery.

According to the National Science Foundation, an average person has about twelve thousand to sixty thousand thoughts per day. Of those, eighty percent are negative, and ninety five percent are repetitive thoughts. If we repeat those negative thoughts, we think negative way more than we think positive. To reiterate, we are what we think. Our thoughts become our reality. That reality can affect our mental health. The condition of our mental health, if unhealthy, can retrogress and develop into mental illness. Learning how to defend thoughts that did not serve the greater good of my mindset, improved the level of my mentality. The command of my thoughts led to proper decision making. Proper decision making evolved into better behaviors. These behaviors redesigned and strengthened healthy mental habits. The way of the warrior would be my line of self-defense in protecting the state of my mental health. Keeping myself present in the moment and always virtuous when met with a threat to my mental health. An exercise that can be done daily that will break the habit of negative thinking that I found worked extremely well, was to write down all my negative thoughts such as insecurities, trust issues, fears, things I did not like about other people etc... and then I would write out at least one positive thought that countered the negative one. If I feared failure, I would write about how failure taught me a valuable lesson in which I was able to benefit from. If I wrote a negative thing about someone's personality, I would write a couple positive things about them that I liked. If I had insecurity about my capability, I would write about all the growth I had gone through since the beginning of the process. Repeating this everyday created a new habit that my mind and brain recognized and remembered. Slowly forming a new subconscious habit. A positive thought enabling habit that truly bettered my mindset and enriched the state of my mental health. Mastering being able to absorb any thought without having to accept it.

I had always worked out physically and it would help me feel better. Sometimes that feeling would last all day. Riding it like a wave. Other times the mental rewards unfortunately did not always stay with me. Depending on environmental factors, all the positive energy could dissipate quickly when met with adversity. When I supplemented strength conditioning in the form of brain exercises into my workout routine, I was able to train my brain and body at the same time. Improving brain function, which not only enhanced the state of my mind but also improved my performance physically. A clear and focused mind and body is capable of anything. Being in a harmonious balance excelled the level of my brain and body fitness. Physical activity raises the heart rate and that increases the flow of blood to the brain. As we work harder, our breathing elevates and pumps additional amounts of oxygen into our bloodstream, which means more oxygen is transported to the brain. This leads to neurogenesis which is the production of neurons. These neurons, depending on what part of the brain, control thinking and memory. One of the side effects of depression and anxiety is memory loss and compromised short term memory, so this increased brain volume and cognitive activity could be helpful in reversing the effects of that. The same could be said perhaps for dementia.

Adding the dedication to learning new subjects, new material, problem solving, writing, painting, creating, all together brought the level of my brain function to a new height. United with enhanced biochemical production from physical exercise the state of my mind was more capable than ever. Through meditation I gained the ability to defend the over clustering of my mind that previously had an impact on my mental health. Becoming deliberate with my thoughts by being intentional and integral with them. Having the courage to think without fear. Letting the thoughts be that served no purpose to me anymore. Respecting my thoughts and myself. Being honest with myself about my thoughts, so that I could properly understand their origin and how to navigate them. Honoring the experiences from the past as lessons but staying present minded in the moment. Remaining loyal to myself and to maintaining the state of positive mental health no matter what. This practice of mental self-defense would also contribute to the harmonious balance of mind and body. Being in this amicable relationship with the brain, the mind and the body was prolific in my recovery and established the new standard routine for my continued success. There is absolutely no doubt in my mind whatsoever that the combination of exercising these three crucial elements of health collectively produced significantly improved results in my mood, sleeping patterns, daily life, overall happiness and directly and dramatically emphatically influenced the shape of my mental health. Efficiently neutralizing my depression and allowing me to finally take off my suit of armor. I am not stating that this is the be all and end all cure for mental illness, specifically depression. I am saying that this worked for me and may just be a natural remedy that might work for you.

Remember, your mind is your best weapon

.

CHAPTER 17

REARVIEW MIRROR

A bend in the road is not the end of the road...unless you fail to make the turn.
Helen Keller

For so long in my life, I had been driving down the only road I had ever been down. Constantly looking in the rearview mirror as I drove on. Blind to my surroundings and the onward scope. I was so preoccupied with what I saw that was behind me, I did not take the time to look ahead. Focused on that rearview mirror. I missed tremendous amounts of turn offs and roads along the way in which I could have traveled down. Ignoring opportunities for a new route. Roads that could have introduced me to new freedoms, new friends, new life. Instead, I stayed on the only road I've ever known. Scared of what lay ahead. Every day, looking back in the rearview mirror to see how far from nowhere I had gone. Starting in the same spot and ending up at the end of the road. Destined to eternally repeat. Fueled by regret. The driving force of my unhappiness. The comfort of the same road travelled I suppose one could say even though it was always an uncomfortable ride. My eyes deadlocked in that rearview mirror.

It wasn't until the day that I closed my eyes and let go of the steering wheel that I crashed in the intersection where my life as I knew it was to die and the birth of a new one was born. It was there that I climbed from the wreckage and looked onward to the frontline of a new frontier. Although badly damaged and severely injured, I found a new road that took me home. A place I had never been before. It was right in front of me the whole time.

Suicide is often referred to as a permanent solution for a temporary problem. Temporary is an indefinite agonizing duration of time for someone with depression or in a depressed state of mental health, like me, temporary can seem like an eternity. An inescapable amount of time. Depression has the capability to strip away hope and reality and replace it with deception and distortion. The deeper the hole dug by depression in the mind, the more difficult it becomes to see anything but the hole you are in. Fixating on being trapped inside the hole without a way out instead of seeing a way to climb out. It is like slowly getting buried alive as the hole gets deeper. Or at least the hole is perceived to get deeper. That is what depression does. Depression impedes the cognitive capability to help yourself or ask for help. Many people, if stuck in a hole would call out for help instantly and in the meantime, they would also begin to attempt to find a way to get out on their own, until help arrived. Not giving up until they found a way out. A person with depression is significantly less likely to call out for help because they do not want to burden anyone else with their problems. As well, feelings of shame and guilt overtake the mind making it very laborious to ask for help. This adds to the dislocation from oneself and others, intensifying the amplification of feeling utterly all alone and having no way out. Now imagine being stuck in that hole for a month inside your mind. The distortion of reality is that you cannot climb out and the deception is that you will never climb out.

Albert Einstein said, "We cannot solve our problems with the same thinking we used when we created them. "The same can be said about the state of the mind. Or the state of the health of mind. To solve the problem of getting out of the hole created by the depressed mind is to change the state of mind. Easier said than done. The psychological and physiological behaviors profoundly change because of being trapped in the hole for so long. Becoming more reclusive and withdrawn from the world around you. Disrupting energy levels make you feel low and weak. So, being mentally, emotionally, and physically weakened only contributes to the draining sense of hopelessness incurred during an episode of depression. Essentially making the hole feel deeper than it is and that there is absolutely no way out. Being trapped in the hole becomes a new reality. From the outside looking in, it is delusional, but not so much for someone with severe depression. The only thing that keeps you company is the pain of your suffering. This suffering acts like blinders on a racehorse sprinting towards only the finish that the blinders allow it to see. Narrow vision creates narrow mindedness. Making everything else nonexistent and inconsequential. This is how suicidal ideation begins.

When I was suicidal, I did not want to die or end my life. In fact, I was terrified of death. I wanted to end the pain and anguish of my life. I had become so unrecognizably delusional to reality. The anomalous combination of my ego pushing me towards suicide in an esoteric attempt of the self-preservation of my image of identity accompanied by the looping cycle of pain from my depression that I felt, became lethal together. I saw no other way out. Blind to reason and rationale. The only future I was capable of seeing was one where I was completely alone. Alone to suffer with all my pain. My ego destroyed my self-esteem by flooding my mind with a never-ending onslaught of the worst selection of my failures, humiliations, and heartbreaks. Causing the inability to navigate my thoughts properly and empower the negative doomsday outcome in any visions of hope that I had. My depression and obsessive thought behavior centered around all the pain from my past. I created scenarios over and over in my mind until I had literally convinced myself that what I was imagining was real. It is like watching the same movie over and over again, except every time the plot becomes more dismal and darker. The ending becomes pessimistically more tragic. Until the movie materializes into the epitome of bitterness and sorrow. The main character dies slowly and painfully. Sucking you deeper into its artificial internal conspiracy that it becomes a vortex in which you cannot escape. Not a fun movie to watch. Imagine having the lead role.

I believe that my exposure to suicide as a young boy and my attempt at it early in my life has always been the tapestry in which my suicidal ideation flourished. Perhaps always keeping it in my back pocket as a solution to escape my depression throughout my life. While trapped inside the vicious cycle of my depression I would think and talk very negatively to myself about myself. Always putting myself down. Condemning myself for never being a success. For not being like other people. Never fitting in anywhere. I knew that many people had or did love me, but it mattered nothing to me because I was unable to feel it. I steadily created negative scenarios by negative fortune telling. Predicting unhappiness and failure in my future based on what had happened to me in the past. I beat myself up from the moment I opened my eyes. My brain became addicted to the hard wiring I was generating. Responding with stress hormones that hindered the production of serotonin and dopamine as well as other neurotransmitters. Drinking alcohol daily was the catalyst for more brain damage and depression-like symptoms as well as additional damage to the deterioration of my physical health. My responses to any emotional stimuli had become increasingly negatively exaggerated. I met anything new with bitterness and discontent. Utter disheartenment.

Shame, guilt, and apathy weakened my emotional state. The shame of never living up to what others wanted from me or for what I wanted for myself, the humiliation that comes with that. The guilt of hurting myself and other people all my life. The apathetic behavior of being emotionless and calloused. Losing everything that I loved and treasured.

Depression runs in my family. Making me genetically dispositioned to it. The extremities of my traumas in my younger years and my wild and out of control lifestyle had been strong environmental contributors. Physical, sexual, and emotional abuse. Torture. Abandonment. Years of drug and alcohol use. Bullying. Violence. Living my life as though I did not care whether I lived or died. Self-destruction. A collaboration of all the misses and falls in my personal life added to the mix with the external influences that triggered tipping points emotionally for me.

Leading up to November 19th, 2019, when it all came crashing down. I could no longer play the comedian. The clown had run out of gimmicks. No disguises that could not be seen through. No more lies. The actor in me could no longer pretend. What started slowly over the few years before that day began to snowball and pickup speed overtime. With that speed came momentum. That momentum created force. My depression went from typically lasting a couple days to a week, to a month, then to a year. Then enter suicidal ideation as the way out of the hole. A nihilistic mindset. The annihilation of my immobilized conscious self. As I continually battered myself for feeling this way it gave strength and fortified the reasoning to end my life. A cruel and violent way to escape. A sadistic subconscious way of punishing myself for giving up, I suppose. Paradoxical madness.

I knew what I was doing was wrong, but it did not matter enough to stop me in the moments leading up to my suicide attempt. My mind had convinced myself that there was no other way. The state of my mental health was so deteriorated at that time that I believed I would be doing the world a favor by dying. My ego wanted to make sure that I would be remembered as the person that looked like they had it all, preserving that image of me indefinitely. I was completely absorbed in a selfish yet helpless disposition. The mind is the most powerful thing, and that power can be very dangerous when manipulated by Mental Illness or a weakened state of mental health. Similar to a puppeteer pulling on the strings that control the animated actions of the puppet. If the strings are pulled on relentlessly too hard and for too long, they snap, losing control of the puppet and the puppet show is then over.

As human beings we often are too late to the revelation of awareness of our mind awakening. It often takes tragic experiences to open up our eyes. This was assuredly the case for me.

In the fresh moments after I had regained somewhat of my composure realizing that I had failed in my attempt to take my life, I was immediately besieged with guilt and shame. There was a small little feeling of relief, but I was not able to focus on that. I was caught up in what felt like being lost in a forest. I was trying to find bearings and direction while anxious thoughts created a fog making it strenuous to navigate. I knew I could find my way out of the forest. I just needed to calm down and breathe.

When I look back, it was in that enigmatic moment that I concluded that the universe had composed a thoroughly different proposition other than what I had for myself. Exposing the true nature of my own fear of living my life within that moment where I should have been dead. It would take the feeling of losing my life to finally understand why I should live. What I mean by that is I had always held myself back from truly living my life due to fear and the attachment of the accompanying hardwiring bad habits which disables self-belief. I had been slowly and gradually killing the life from myself. A slow burn suicide over my lifetime. Everything suddenly made sense amidst the most chaotic moment of my life. I finally had found something to die for. Which in turn made me want to live more. I know that sounds backwards, but it could not be more accurate in my case. My purpose was given to me at that moment through the instinctive fight or flight response. I either fought for my life and would share my experience to help educate and influence the minds of anyone else who was in a struggle with their own lives, or I gave up and ended my life.

What appeared to be the weakest point of my life became the strongest. I would use that newfound strength to push through the next few months. Creating a battle system to outwit the enemies on the battleground inside my head. I needed to outsmart my own brain and take control of my mind. To do that, I had to go back to the start. Where all my thought habits and patterns began. I would face all the traumatic experiences starting from my early childhood to the present. I had to comprehend the dynamics of these events and trace back all the associated feelings and emotions attached to the memories to become truly aware of them. If I could travel back to the origins of these issues and understand how they shaped my behavior, then I could devise a new formula to change them. Constituting a growth plan. This hypothesis over the next few months would determine astonishing results in not only deconstructing my recurring suicidal ideation but would also be critical in dismantling and taking down the walls inside the constructs of my depression. Freeing my mind from the prison cell that my negative thought patterns and habits had so unkindly designed for me. It would seem that we are all prisoners inside our own cages that we design ourselves. Sadly, the door is wide open, or the key is in our pocket and all we must do is take that first step and walk out into the unknown. For myself, it took nearly dying to come legitimately and honestly to understand who I was and why I behaved the way I did. I am now in a constant state of perpetual learning every day and am a student of my own life. I remain in an uninterrupted adaptive and evolving mindset that is fluid and can take many shapes and forms like water. Becoming the best fit for whatever position my internal and external surroundings permit. My symptoms from my various Mental Illnesses are still there and will always have an involvement in my life. By learning from all my experiences, I was able to recognize and diagnose triggers and tipping points that had previously been able to sway my direction or halt my momentum. I designed a chart-like model to do this as I am a very visual pupil. The basis of the model was to illustrate the event or experience that had had a traumatic imprint on my life and trace the thoughts, feelings, emotions, and behaviors from that and connect them to the appropriate Mental Illness or state of my mental health. Administering a tangible representation of the connections between all the specific details involved. What became important was being able to identify the root or core of the involvement of the established cause and then following the sequence of events from that. This allowed me to study the patterns of how my experiences shaped my behavior. The relevance of all this is that it exposed a recognizable template which I could reference and sight in making my battle system and growth plan. Enabling comprehension of triggers and tipping points so that I could successfully self-defend against similar present or future experiences. Answering what, when, why, where, and how, I became more knowledgeable about myself, and knowledge is power according to GI Joe.

On the flipside, I would expose the same traumatic incident but chart the positive direction from it in the exact same way as I did the negatives. The findings were fascinating to me because it exhibited the total opposite results. Giving me clear indication that the data was the same but the landscape of my thoughts, feelings, emotions, and behaviors totally changed in the most profound manner. Basically, showcasing the experience had a dual purpose in shaping my personality traits as in behaviors and habits. I had the opportunity to choose which perspective to take based on this model. I could either focus my energy wallowing in the past and staying in a depressed mindset or I could focus my energy on the present moment and use my successes from these failures to empower my actions towards growth. This model is a system that can be used to alter habits. Our daily habits are what make us or break us. Every small habit that is changed for the objective of learning, improving, and growing becomes easier once the removal of the bad habit that impedes this happens. Through recognition of the original source of the bad habit sighted in this model, I could use it as a reference point to register my progress when challenged with new experiences that had the potential to trigger negative reactions in my mind. This way I could systematically identify when and why my mind started to wander in the wrong direction or become overwhelmed with spinning thoughts and chart my way back by using the positive reinforcement illustrated on the model. Simplifying instead of complexifying the process. Overthinking leads unquestionably nowhere quickly, a destination I was far too familiar with previously in my life. This universal model can be used for combat with any Mental Illness, Mental Health issue or any situation that is causing interruption and difficulty in life. Taking the extra few minutes when facing bad thought habits and changing them judiciously by using this model has helped me to transform into a wiser and understanding version of myself. Self-acceptance and self-efficacy continue to increase, and I appreciate every experience as a favorable circumstance to learn more about myself and how to eliminate shame and guilt by forgiving, respecting, and loving the person I have fought hard to become.

Depression is a very lonely road that can lead nowhere or to the end of the road. Suicide is the end of the road. Every person in this world has a unique and extraordinary story about their experiences in life. Just because someone has what looks like a fascinating and fantastic life does not mean that they are immune to winding up lost on the road alone with nowhere to go. Losing their way home. I am living proof of this.

My biggest regret is that I did not ask for help when I needed it the most. I ignored the people around me that loved me and wanted to help. It could have prevented me from leaving it to chance or fate to still be alive today. The odds of a firearm jamming according to Google are one in nine hundred to one thousand rounds. Being what should have been the first round fired, I am somehow still here against all odds.

If anyone is having thoughts of suicide, please talk to someone immediately. Call your friends, your family or contact the suicide prevention resources available in your area. Please do not make the same mistakes I made and understand that there is hope. There is a way out of the hole no matter how deep it has become. You are not alone and there are people that care about you. We are different but also all the same, we may have different circumstances, situations, and events in our lives, but we are connected through our struggles and our triumphs together. The world is a more beautiful place because we are in it. Whatever we are going through is temporary no matter how hard it is. When we rebuild ourselves from the broken fragments of our despair, we become beautiful and bright. We can become light for others in darkness. A symbol of strength. I believe in you. I want to hear your stories. I want you to shine so bright that the shadows have nowhere to hide.

If someone you know is struggling with depression or suicide, please be that person that goes beyond checking in. There are Suicide Prevention Support resources available. Be relentless in your pursuit to help. Provide safety and comfort. Listen but ask the hard questions in a compassionate way. Depression and Suicide are often concealed through self-isolation masked as many other things as possible like being tired, sick, or not feeling oneself. Behaviors to watch for are:

*Increased substance abuse- alcohol, drugs, pills
*Dramatic mood changes
*Feelings of being trapped, like there is no way out
*Anxiety, increased agitation, and uncontrollable anger
*Feelings of hopelessness and helplessness, having no purpose in life
*Sudden withdrawal from friends, family, work, and general society
*Insomnia, or sleeping all the time
*Living recklessly without caring

The smallest gesture of kindness can be the determining fact of either life or death for someone contemplating suicide. Let me share a story about that.

Many years ago, I was riding my motorcycle on the highway after a very hot Manitoba summer day. It was early in the evening. I was headed towards Winnipeg, returning from a small town south of the city after visiting an old biker friend. Being in the prairies I could see for kilometers ahead of where I was travelling. Although it had been a very hot and sunny day, in the horizon I could clearly see a severe thunderstorm developing very rapidly. Huge dark grey cumulonimbus clouds that were conjugating together forming a wall across the sky. The clouds moved in circles above and below each other in a war between cold and warm air masses. As I sped towards the storm on my motorcycle suddenly the temperature dropped considerably as did the air pressure. The winds began to pick up and were blowing their might against me. As I neared the perimeter of the storm clouds, I noticed that some of the clouds had gotten so dark that the grey had a green and dark purple tone to it. At that moment the clouds dropped and looked as though they were almost touching the ground ahead of me. Lightning and thunder erupted all around me and then came the punishing rains. It started pouring huge cold raindrops that were pelting and pummeling as they hit me. I leaned down closely to my motorcycle and pinned it, accelerated into the storm to try, and break through it before it got worse. I was wearing a small beanie style helmet which protected the top of my head, but not my face, a leather vest over a t-shirt and jeans which provided no safety from the impact of those raindrops that felt like someone was stabbing me all over with a blunt knife on my exposed skin. The clouds above were forming funnel clouds as I got closer to the center of the storm. Funnel clouds can turn into tornadoes, so my adrenaline was skyrocketing. A few seconds later the rain was coming down so hard I could no longer see twenty feet in front of me, like a sheet of water. Then it went from very bad to even worse. Hail.

I needed to find shelter immediately. The hailstones were the size of grapes and felt like bullets when they hit my body. I was in real danger as my skin was being split open on my hands and arms from the impact of the hail. I was losing visibility and would soon not be able to handle my motorcycle. I was in the middle of nowhere. I was screaming in pain inside my mind. Out of nowhere appeared a very small house with a light on just off the highway. Just as I slowed down and was making the turn to go towards the house a Semi truck barreled past, unable to see me in the rain and hail just missing the back wheel of my motorcycle by mere inches. I made my way down the gravel driveway that was flooded from the rain to the small house and took refuge inside the carport. Winds were increasing, lightning and thunder struck what seemed like every second and the storm was intensifying. After taking a moment to calm myself, shaking off the insanity I was wearing all over me from the storm. I walked over to the door on the side of the house that was covered by the carport. The top half of the door had a clear glass insert that was slid half open halfway and I could see inside. I looked around and I saw a man sitting in a chair watching television. He was watching Sixty Minutes. A great show with riveting content and investigative reporting. I was sure he must have heard the roar of my Harley as I pulled up in his carport but perhaps the continuous growling thunder had drained it out. I knocked on the glass window of the door, but the man did not move. I noticed he had a glass in one hand that looked like it had whiskey in it. I knocked again, this time louder. He still did not move. I thought to myself "what the heck man!" So, I pounded on the door and this time he finally moved. He barked at me and told me to go away. I explained to him loudly that I could not do that because of the extreme storm outside. I told him about my situation and asked him if he had an old jacket and a pair of work gloves, I could use to cover myself from the hail and rain so I could attempt to ride through the storm to get home, as the storm showed no sign of letting up. I told him I was stuck there and needed his help. He lowered his chin to his chest and looked like he took a deep pensive breath. He had not even turned around to see who was at his door which I found puzzling. He slowly stood up, took a long look at the television, put his drink down on the side table and then finally turned to face me. I saw a large man, tall with dark short hair. He reminded me a little bit of Frankenstein dressed in a classic farmer's sense of style. He had dark circles under his eyes even though his face was very tanned from the summer sun. His eyes looked lifeless as he walked towards me. He did not say a word as he walked past the door. He returned momentarily with a pair of leather work gloves and a red and black plaid lumber jacket. He opened the door and held them out for me to take. I thanked him and told him that I would return them to him the next day. He shrugged and said it was fine and he did not need them back. Then he just stood there silent and motionless for a couple seconds. I asked him if he was ok if something was wrong? He shook his head slightly and said he was fine. I asked him what his name was, and he seemed quite taken back by that. We will call him Walter; I told him my name and went to shake his hand. I invited myself in for a quick whiskey to warm up from being drenched and then said I would be on my way. As I stepped inside his home, I noticed a shotgun leaning against the chair he was sitting in. I remember thinking to myself that he probably grabbed it when he heard my motorcycle pull up. Bikers sometimes can have bad reputations. I pretended I didn't see it. He poured me a whiskey and grabbed his glass, and we had a quick drink together. We did not say much. I talked about the intensity of the storm. I asked him again if he was alright and he replied yes. I was not convinced that he was ok. I looked Walter in the eyes, and I asked him this. "What do you call a fake noodle?" He looked at me like he was quite confused. I replied "An im-pasta" There was a brief second of very awkward silence and then we both cracked up laughing hysterically. His face totally changed. It lit up. Nothing like a bad joke to break the ice. I shook his hand and slapped him on the shoulder, thanking him on my way out the door. I put on my newly acquired gear and started up my Harley and back into the storm I rode. It took about fifteen excruciating minutes that felt like hours to finally break through the storm. Thanks to Walter, I made it home safe. I was banged up and bruised, welts and cuts all over my face and body from the hail, my tanks and fenders on my bike had been dimpled and dented from the hail as well. All repairable. His kindness went a long way with me. For the record I will say that Walter had the weirdest and creepiest laugh I had ever heard.

I drove out the next day and returned Walter's things. He was not there when I arrived, so I left them on top of a wood pile just inside the carport. With a note inside the front pocket that said "im-pasta"

Flash forward to several years later I was visiting a friend who had checked herself into rehab in Winnipeg. She was admitted into an intake program and was allowed visitors during her recovery. Visitation took place in an open cafeteria like setting with bright lighting. We were chatting away when I noticed a man across the room was looking at me. I continued talking with my friend and every time I looked up, that man was still looking at me, this time he was smiling at me. I asked my friend if she knew who the guy was, and she told me that he worked there. He was an addictions counselor. I thought to myself he probably thinks I'm an alcoholic or addict. He would be right. As our visit ended the man walked over to me as I was about to leave. He asked if he could have a quick word with me and I assumed he wanted to ask how my visit went. He said he would walk with me outside. Once we were outside the building, he turned to me and smiled from ear to ear and asked me "what do you call a fake noodle?" "An im-pasta" he said as he broke out in hysterical laughter. The weirdest creepiest laughter I had ever heard. It was Walter and I did not even recognize him. He looked so different. I was in shock. He gave me a big hug and told me that he was so happy to see me. He went on to tell me that the day before the storm his wife had left him because of his out-of-control drinking. That he was watching sixty minutes because it was their favorite show to watch together. He told me that at the end of the show when the stopwatch stopped ticking, that he was going to shoot himself, but I showed up out of nowhere in the middle of a thunderstorm and interrupted that. My company and my joke were enough to disrupt his plan of suicide that night. He told me that he believed that my visit was a sign for him not to commit suicide. The next day he checked himself into rehab. Once sober, he sold his farm property and went back to school and became an addictions counselor so he could help other people just like him. We chatted for a while and then he had to return to work. It was such an amazing story that I was totally bewildered by. My mind was blown. What are the chances of that? According to the magic of the universe there are no chances or coincidences. Only that the smallest gesture of kindness is the conductor of the biggest miracles. Good thing I wasn't looking in my rearview mirror on that highway.

It is no longer possible to fear the darkness when you become a source of light that guides others through it.

CHAPTER 18

THE ALMIGHTY WATERFALL

A waterfall begins with one drop of water sir, look what comes from that...
from the book The Power of One

A waterfall is a beautiful and powerful thing. A true wonder of nature. Captivating and breathtaking. Magical. It is a body of water that falls over a rocky edge into a pool below. Some waterfalls are massive where water cascades down hundreds of meters. In fact, the tallest waterfall in the world is called Angel Falls found in Venezuela and it is a ginormous three thousand and twelve feet or nine hundred and seventy-nine meters high. It is fifteen times taller than Niagara Falls. When its water is plentiful in the wet season tiny water drops can be felt from it as far as one kilometer away. Sometimes it splits into two waterfalls as well. On the flipside, waterfalls can be small too. Often called cascades, these waterfalls are smaller in height and lesser in their steepness and often form a series of small falls. Waterfalls range in size, strength and are located all over the globe. Always a worthwhile adventure, seeking out waterfalls and the hike to get to them is often a physically and mentally advantageous journey.

Waterfalls often form as rivers or streams progress from soft rock to hard rock. This happens laterally as the streams flow across the surface and vertically as the water drops in a waterfall. This creates erosion of the soft rock exposing a harder ledge which from the river falls. The process of erosion is that of wearing away earth. This process is fundamental in the formation of a waterfall. Waterfalls themselves are a contributing factor in erosion. As the water continues to flow, it picks up and carries sediment. Depending on the size of the stream or river, it could be microscopic silt, pebbles, or even big old boulders. This sediment erodes the riverbeds made of sandstone or limestone or other soft rock, steepening its grade. Over time, that exposes a hard rock like granite or dolomite which remains less affected by erosion. Waterfalls then develop as these granite rock formations form cliffs and ledges. The river's velocity dramatically increases as it funnels near the site of the waterfall which escalates the amount of erosion that takes place. Creating smooth flattened rocks. The rushing water and its contained sediments topple over the waterfall, eroding any surface it touches on the way down as well as eroding the plunge pool it forms at its base. The force of the crashing water can create whirlpools that further erode of the existing pools. This can cause water to recess behind where the waterfall is, creating a cave behind it. There are other contributing factors that can create waterfalls in nature outside of geology and erosion. Tectonic movement drops in sea level, and glaciers have all had their part in the history of formation of waterfalls around the world.

A waterfall is a symbol of ecological health. They indicate a healthy ecosystem when the stream of water is consistently ample and healthy which is reflected in the abundance of life in the area surrounding it. As they flow into different streams and rivers, waterfalls purify the water. Purification of water establishes the healthy stock of oxygen that the diverse aquatic life depends on to live. Further enhancing the ecosystem.

All of this is compelling and rich information but there exist even more exciting reasons why waterfalls are so attractive. Waterfalls stimulate three senses simultaneously which also flirts with some of our primordial instincts. Sight, hearing, and smell are all positively aroused when in the presence of the almighty waterfall.

The intoxicating effect we feel when we see a waterfall is the raw natural beauty of it combined with the fact that its unremitting flow is ever changing which challenges one of our purposes of sight which is to identify patterns in what we see. This is exhilarating and our brains love it. Graceful in its flow, it can be captivating. Presenting a feeling of reassurance from the chaotic world. Giving us the sense of connection to nature that emphasizes a feeling of being more alive. The hypnotic crashing water causes a rainbow mist that is stunning and adds to the overall stimuli of the experience.

A waterfall is often heard before it is seen. This gets the blood pumping in anticipation of discovering the waterfall. A massive fall can be as loud as a jet engine, or in some cases even louder. The roaring of the falling water and rapids creates a calming yet thrilling sensation as we hear it. A smaller waterfall may produce a gentle trickle that eases the mind. Either way, making it possible to hear the waterfall just as much as seeing the waterfall.

The smell of a waterfall is alluring and tantalizes with its ultimate scent of freshness. Like the smell of a recent rainfall, clean and fresh water falls in the form of vapor and this propositions our primal instinctive nature of invariably seeking out fresh water for survival. But wait, there is more.

Waterfalls release negative ions. In this particular case, being negative is a positive thing. The crashing waters from a waterfall generate a profusion of negative ions hidden in the fast-moving waters and the vapor being produced by them. A negative ion is an oxygen atom that has picked up an extra electron giving it a negative charge. Invisible to the human eye, they are launched into the air and are powerfully dynamic. Breathing them in immediately begins to recharge our batteries. As we soak the negative ions in, and they reach our bloodstream the production of serotonin is increased. We get a natural boost that reduces anxiety and depression while invigorating energy and happiness. The negative ions released from waterfalls can also positively affect metabolism, immune system, digestion, blood pressure, sleep patterns and overall emotional states. All these astounding sensations just from being in the presence of a waterfall.

Wherever I have travelled throughout my life I have made sure to set out on an adventure to find any nearby waterfalls if geographically possible. Never once being disappointed with what I discovered. I have often found myself marveling in the magnificence of a waterfall whether its presence was peaceful or powerful. Sitting there for hours absorbing its energies. Cleansing. Detoxifying. The combined stimulations are so strong that it literally pushes out all other thoughts and feelings from the mind. Being situated in the natural beauty of its raw setting is freeing and rejuvenating. When possible, swimming in the plunge pool provided by the falls, exploring behind the waterfall, allowing the waterfall to shower over me, and surveying the area around it for its biological diversity has been so therapeutic and healing for me on so many assorted mental and emotional levels. Always on the lookout for frogs. Breathing in the clean air, reflecting on the challenges of the trek to get to the waterfall sets a positive state of mental health and physical well-being. The connection to nature has always been a grounding guiding force in my life. Bringing me back to the simplest singular thoughts with gigantic complex potentials. Proportional to the fact that the almighty roaring waterfall started with just a singular drop of water. Big things have small beginnings.

Can one person change the world? Can I be that one person? Can you be that one person? Can one idea change the world? The answer is a gigantic, enormous pink and blue neon sign the size of a city with millions of fireworks exploding behind it in the sky that screams YES!

I believe that we all have the power to change the world around us with everything we do because everything is connected by the very fact that we are all alive right now in this moment together. That alone is an astronomical miracle. That is magic. It is up to every individual to find their own magic and use it to put on a show for the world to see. Captivating those around you with the story behind finding your magic because it never comes from somewhere, it comes from someone. That someone is you. But something must happen for your magic to come to life. That something is unique to each person. For many people it comes from the moment that we decide to make a change. When we take action. It often originates from our most desperate and painful moments. When we finally decide to face our fear of the unknown and fight back against it, making a change in our lives for the better, is when the magic begins. One punch at a time. One step at a time. Or in the case of a waterfall, one drop of water at a time.

If we are to compare changing our actions one at a time with consistency to that of drops of water corresponding to creating a waterfall, it reveals a constant flow of movement carving through the hard parts which erodes a path that can be followed. The point of this illustration is that if a waterfall can start with one drop of water that begins the sequence of events that follow it, so too can you do the same metaphorically speaking with one step in a new direction of one action. Start moving and make a path. The next step becomes easier, less friction, smoother transitions. And so on and so on. Like a waterfall. The bigger the waterfall the more powerful it becomes, just like a person with a purpose. A waterfall is attractive and awe inspiring by its energy, poise, balance of peacefulness and power and its natural raw beauty. Captivating those in its presence. A person is no different. When a person becomes like a waterfall the people around them begin to feel better. Just like the ions that are released by the fast-moving waters of a waterfall, people give off positive vibes when they are in a true genuine state of fluidity of harmonious, powerful, and peaceful thought. Meaning that when a person is true to themselves, they are not trying but just doing, becoming a beacon of inspiration just like a waterfall to others around them. Magnetism. What is surrounding them grows because of this. This is where the magic comes into play. Becoming that first drop of water and creating a new waterfall is life changing. Not just your own life changes but changes other lives around you. The direct influence by leading change helps in the erosion of our illusions of fear and failure. By sharing our stories, we can erode the stigma and become a powerful and inspirational force like a waterfall together. The more we share the more powerful we become as people who have lost their way due to mental illness or sickness can hear the roar of the voice of the waterfall. See the change in the patterns of the minds that had been constricted by fear of failure and judgement as the waters continually pound upon those hardened minds until they become smoother and accepting. A waterfall is relentless in its contribution to its environment, and we need to sustain this action as well in our daily activities.

If every single thought is connected to all the other thoughts in my mind, and I am able to connect an emotion to that single new thought by attaching an action to it. I believe that this causes the other thoughts in my mind to sway in the direction of the feeling initialized by the change in activity. Positively influencing the chain reaction of events to follow in my mind. I also believe that this contagious waterfall-like premise can flow through the connections made by being bold and courageous in sharing the stories in which the magic breakthrough moment in our lives happens and how we got there. Magic is often referred to when an event takes place that is unexplainable, wonderful, unexpected and that supernatural powers could be at play. Making things appear or disappear or perhaps controlling events in nature are the results of magic. That is why I believe in magic. I believe that if one drop of water can start a waterfall then one thought creates an action that can start a new life, then I believe that one idea has the magical capability of changing the entire world. That idea is sharing my story. Making the stigma plaguing mental illness disappear, unconditional understanding of mental illness appears, creating the waterfall effect that can change lives as each drop of water flows forward generating direction and leadership for those in need. The inclusive connections we all share are influential in the inspiration for ourselves and others. I am an almighty waterfall and so are you.

Now I do enjoy the music of TLC just as much as anyone else. They had some great jams back in the day, there is no doubt about that. One of their biggest hits was a song titled "Don't Go Chasing Waterfalls." However, I strongly disagree with the lyrics of the chorus and do advise that you do go chasing waterfalls and please do not stick to the rivers and lakes that you are used to. There are literally thousands of waterfalls in Canada and millions of waterfalls worldwide. The continent of Europe has the largest concentration of waterfalls, and the country of Norway has the most waterfalls of any other country in the world. The city of Hamilton in Ontario, Canada which is located on the banks of the great Lake Ontario is home to one hundred and fifty-six waterfalls within its city limits making it the city with the most waterfalls in the entire world.

Explore whenever and wherever you can, go chase those waterfalls literally and figuratively. You might just become one yourself amid the journey and adventure. Becoming that magical one drop of water that starts it all.

CHAPTER 19

THE BEGINNING

When writing the story of your life, do not let anyone else hold the pen.
Harley Davidson

Every day that I worked on this book, my mind told me to quit. That people would not like what I have written that they will not understand my message. My mind told me every day that I was not good enough to have the right to share my story. That people will laugh at me. Every day I was faced with the choice to either quit or persist and carry on moving forward. Somedays I moved slowly like a snail. Other days, I broke down and I cried while I wrote. Sometimes I screamed and got up and had a temper tantrum like a child because I could not find the right words to express what I was attempting to say. I would lose track of where I was in the story, forgetting where I was going with my ideas. There were times when I rewrote the same thing a hundred different ways until I liked how it was worded. The voice in my head told me to stop. While following my dream to be an author I lost everything. My job. My vehicle. I had absolutely no money. I had to borrow. This would have usually set me off the tracks, but I had discovered something more valuable than that inside myself. I had a purpose, and

I made the commitment to that purpose so I could help other people like me or like you. Somedays I laughed out loud at myself. I read out loud to all my houseplants that surrounded me every single time I wrote. Having full out conversations with them at times. I got up and danced like a fool. I cried happy tears when I completed the real gut punching material. I fantasized about hurling my laptop like a discus across the sky all the way from Winnipeg to over the mountains in British Columbia. There were days that I thought I was losing my mind, there were days that I did not want to find it. I will always face the challenges of my mental Illnesses but through self-discipline and dedication, I always pushed forward. Taking that first step no matter how hard. Once I began to believe in myself and my purpose, I felt like I belonged somewhere. I was humbled in the process of growth. Everything became connected. Associated. In the moment where I should have died, I was given a second chance. Within that chance I found out that I feared living to my potential and had hidden behind fear my whole existence. That had to change. I had to exemplify the embodiment of that change. I believe that by changing my thoughts, that I could change my environment. That would act as a template for others to follow.

When I wanted to give up and give in to fear, I would ask myself this...What if my story reaches someone who was ready to give up. What if that person is a brilliant young mind who was going through similar experiences as I did? What if that beautiful young mind was the person who would accomplish the impossible one day. Creating something that would better the world. Like a beautiful and raw song that reached millions of minds and helped them navigate through difficult times because they could feel it and apply it through relation. Or perhaps that young beautiful mind went on to become a strong leader of a nation that was honest and true to their word and changed the course of history for the greater good. But what if that person did not read this because I chose to give in to fear, and they chose suicide instead because I was too afraid of what people might think of my story and did not follow through on writing this book. That's on me. I owe it to this world and the people in it to share my experience while spinning on this crazy rock we call Earth. I have a responsibility that came with my second chance at life and my story just might give someone else enough hope to get through theirs too. My story just might influence someone to learn more about themselves so they can change their life. That has a ripple effect, and they may influence some they know to better understand Mental illness because someone they love is fighting to stay alive.

Some of us are misplaced in our darkest of darkness. Some of us are trapped in a place we do not want to be because of our depressed mental state of mind related to trauma or tragedy. Some of us are breaking down every day because we are not happy with our lives, our jobs, our spouses/partners, ourselves, but we endure because we are too scared to change. Some of us are chemically imbalanced and cannot comprehend the idea of being able to control our own thoughts and emotional conduct. Some of us pick up the bottle, so we can drink our pain or loneliness away. Some of us are in love with someone who is depressed, bi-polar, anorexic or addicted to a substance and is dying, painstakingly watching our loved ones suffer daily. I don't know exactly what you are going through or how you got there, but I can tell you what can help, because I've been where you are. You need hope. Belief. I want you to know that all of those destroyed damaged pieces of you can become the most beautiful things about you if you don't give up. It is okay to break down, it's okay to cry, it is okay to fall apart into a million little pieces, but it is not okay to give up. I made that mistake and almost lost everything. All the pain, the tears, the desperation of it all, is necessary in the beginning process. You will be sucker punched repeatedly and kicked hard while you are down by all that you fear, early in the process. But that is where the opportunity for our growth comes from. The process will get us closer to where we want to be and, in that process, we will get stronger if we commit to moving forward. Learning to push past our limits by believing in ourselves that we can. We will not always see why or where the process is guiding us at times, but we just need to trust, keep moving until we break through. Once we are standing on our own two feet on the other side of it all, I promise you this based on what I went through, the times you will look back, will be to chart how far you have come, perhaps to share the triumphs of what was overcome and offer a roadmap to someone else who may be lost in a similar way as we formerly once were.

Life will continue to be hard as biology is unpredictable. Life is an all-powerful miracle that does not take sides. We choose to take a side. There will be hardship, calamity, and mishap. We will lose people we love. Our hearts will be broken. We will be let down inside of our circles. We will be betrayed by the ones we trusted most. We will still fail, but we will be stronger now, smarter, having more internal resources to fall back on. We will get through anything. It's okay if it takes time if it takes longer then we are comfortable with. It is okay to feel all of these things as they are components of life. But we can use the pain as fuel to create a fire that burns all negativity in our perspective. Creating a truly positive state. which will in turn provide us with the courage to believe in ourselves and not to give up. Giving up is no longer an option. On the flipside of all those challenges put in our path in life are the epiphanies, revelations, and magic.

What we become in the process is far more important than the dream. Process creates and exposes our purpose which defeats our past demons enabling us to push forward through any adversity thrown our way. The process in which we have adopted into our daily life will build our character and strengthen our word which defines who we truly are. Self-respect is a guiding force within the integrity of our identity.

We could learn to embrace our hardships as tests of will and determination. A moment of liberty, opening ourselves up and honestly looking at the nakedness of our intentions, deeds and how to positively enhance our surroundings. Relying on the protection of our hard-earned self-discipline to stop repeating bad habits. Having the fearlessness to change the people in our life, to only ones that add to our life. The people that are in line with our path, not those who purposely obstruct it. Remove toxicity in our relationships no matter how hard that is, especially in the relationship with ourselves. By constantly facing our fear with the recognition that it is all a delusional illusion created internally, we then can find an intrepid way to see through it. Whether that is being alone, taking the first step into the unknown or believing in yourself so much, that you just take a leap of faith.

As we continue to move forward no matter the circumstance without making excuses. Excuses are lies we tell ourselves to compromise our direction due to fear of failure or success. Excuses rob us of the rewards of accomplishment that are so imperative for our brain health. Embrace our past experiences as opportunities to learn from and recalibrate our focus aligning newfound determination and an emotional attachment to that. This challenges our prefrontal cortex to create new thoughts which can lead to new behaviors as we take new steps into the unknown with an optimistic approach as we have conquered the fear of failing. A drive fueled by compassion for us and others as we create more positive results within ourselves and in our circles. Acting daily to improve our quality of life for ourselves and those around us. We become brighter as we shine in places in our lives that we never have before. Illuminated the darkness so we can continue to navigate our path even in the darkest of times. As we do that more people will follow our light and want to understand and be a part of this positive energy that has been created. Together we can shine so bright that we begin to light up the entire sky as we connect through sharing our stories, our fall, and our triumphs of spirit. Every real connection creates motion and new energies. Our luminescence will outshine the stigma of mental illness opening new education and understanding of this true and very real global pandemic. Our current state in society wants us to disconnect from each other and dim the lights by setting impossible expectations of life. It wants to use darkness to shadow over what we truly need to be successful in having happiness. Through purpose we can outshine anything together. It is no longer possible to fear the darkness when we become a source of light that guides others through it.

We can be freed of our mental and emotional prison cells, our cages. Changing the game up on the environments that catered to the decomposition of our mental health by no longer living in them. Running wild and free as we were meant to. We simply just need to show each other the way by sharing our stories of freedom, liberation and triumph from our fears, our traumas, our heartbreaks and all the guilt and shame that we previously held on to. To exit the harbors of self-destruction where we anchored for far too long and explore the open waters that are calling us.

We can learn a newfound strength to fulfill our purpose in life just like the Monarch Butterfly. With all odds stacked against it, just like us, we can always find a way to get where we need to be. The Monarch Butterfly also teaches us that there are stages of transformation that do not always look pretty but are a vital necessity. We shed our fear of failure and embrace the challenges of the process which guides us to our destinations. We change directions sometimes and get lost, but we can always find our way back when we have trust in our moral compass. It will always aim us in the proper direction in which to take. We can always get back on track. No matter if the overpowering winds are extreme enough to set us off course or the relentless pelting rain from the monstrous thunderstorms above set us back, we can get through them when we believe that we can. We learn that our purpose is always bigger than we are. Once we find our purpose, we can become an unstoppable juggernaut clearing through all that we let hold us back, no matter how big or small we are. Opening the flight path so others can follow and freely migrate through the skies of the changing seasons of our lives.

Opening our minds like young children and seeing the world and life as big as we did back then. Life seemed so much more immense and astonishing. Mesmerized by wonder. Our thoughts were creative and catalyzed with vivid imaginations of what everything could be. As young children every opportunity was simple, challenges were met with enthusiasm, and we played with other kids. We played as Superheroes, Robots, Ninjas, and everything else under the sun recreating our best renditions of those characters with only a colorful imagination and what was in our surroundings. We could transform our bedrooms, a field, the basement, wherever into whatever scenario and setting accompanied the theme just by believing in our imaginative mind. Our backyards could become a tropical rainforest where we were searching for animals, our bedrooms, a Space Station, a nearby park became a battlefield where the rains poured down and tanks were getting stuck in the deep mud. We could even transform our basement into another world in an undiscovered galaxy. We imagined that the snowbanks we climbed were as gigantic as a mountain range. We imagined fighting dinosaurs or merely escaping the jaws of a shark getting out of a swimming pool. We had lightsaber battles with the leftover cardboard rolls from wrapping paper. We believed it in our young minds so much and then we could see it as though it was real. We played sports, we raced, rode bicycles, gymnastics, dancing, anything with motion as young kids. None of us were the best at it, that did not matter. We just loved to play and have fun. We wiped out, we got cuts and bruises, we got up after we fell, sometimes we cried, sometimes we laughed but we always got up. Most times we went right back to what we were doing like nothing happened. If we did not like what we were playing, we would start playing something different. It really was that simple. We did not try to ruin another child's life because they had a different opinion on something. We got over it and moved on. So as young children we were able to change the patterns of our brains through the power of our imagination, yet as adults we have forgotten how empowering this truly is. We imagine ourselves where we want to be, and we can get there. I believe opening our minds and reconnecting to the fearless and adventurous imaginative state of a child-like mind is where we could all become more successful in doing what makes us happy. After all, happiness is the key to all success. Go catch some frogs, lie on your back in a field and look up at the clouds and shape the metamorphosis of the cloud formations, finger paint, have a ballet in your backyard, have a fashion show, pull out the skateboard, and get back up on your bike no matter how many tries it takes. Look at the world for everything it has, not what it does not.

We must consistently fight the stigma that suffocates any new hope from someone with Mental illness. We must work together, in unity. We must form a line with an unbreakable bond with each other. No more tolerance of those ignorant forces that want to keep us depressed, disconnected, and devastated. We must speak out as loud as we can. Challenge the government's actions. Demand that our governments dedicate more to the Mental health budgets and follow through with their claims of action. Question our workplaces policies to help someone cope with Mental Illness. Bringing attention to understanding how to cope with mental illness should be in all our schools as a class subject to help young minds learn and live. We need to let every human being know that it is not their fault that they went through trauma, were born with neurological damage, have chemically imbalanced brain function or whatever it is jeopardizing the quality of their lives to a point that they need help. Our stories bind us together. Our experiences are fundamental. Connections with those who are lost and require comfort and navigation by following our lead are life changing. Learning to share how we truly feel with each other where judgement is replaced by compassion. We need to listen and look for ways to help those in need. Offer support instead of advice. We need to look out of each other's eyes to see what is going on instead of looking into each other's eyes. Just being there for someone could save their life and save the countless amount of people's grief and pain around them. If we can all learn from one and another, our lives connect on so many levels from molecular to spiritual. We remain humble sharing our stories of overcoming our struggles. We connect on such a deeper level while doing this that it strengthens bonds and creates courage within us. Opening our hearts makes us all stronger, wiser and reaffirms our belief in our purpose. Together we can rewrite our stories in a new narrative so that those with a mental illness or anyone struggling with mental health issues can get help without prejudice and criticism but instead are replaced with understanding and support. So that the new and plentiful resources are made easily available. Through our stories we can aid in educating those who do not understand how serious a pandemic mental illness is in our close circles of friends, our families, our cities, our countries and our world and the catastrophic effects that come with it if we do not act now. We will brighten and light the sky a beautiful new color that will attract more attention than the darkness that it illuminates. Darkness is a necessity that we all must make our way through to see the light. By walking through it together, we can help others see the light at the end of their darkness.

If we are all together then we will hold the hands of those who feel isolated and alone so that they can feel hope. We can become the sonorous voice for those who are voiceless in their silent struggles. We can make the encouragement of people asking for help, getting diagnosed properly accompanied with modern therapy and treatment options the new normal. We can become a global inspiration where we put our mental health first, therefore finding new routines of self-discipline that replace self-destruction, newfound stories of self-respect through learning how to love ourselves and then others, exercises both mentally and physically that continue to challenge and engage new thoughts, behavior, and ultimately new ecosystems within the constructs of our new environments. We can teach the world around us that there is not something wrong with us but are at times clinging to life by a desperate little shred of hope because it's all we have left due to our depression. We can enlighten the minds of those who cannot comprehend that we are dealing with a brain illness that is as life threatening as cancer or heart disease as ninety percent of the suicides in the world are by people with depression. Suicide is a leading cause of death. That if we look at statistics from almost everywhere in the world that suicide is consistently in the top ten causes of death, in some countries it is in the top five. We need to study the long-term effects of depression as it leads to heart disease and shortens the length of life dramatically. If we find new forms of treatment other than pharmaceutical solutions that we greatly improve the quality of life for those with Mental Illness. Exercise, yoga, meditation, reading books, learning new things daily, transcendence of thoughts and feelings, therapy, and sharing our experience with one another are good examples that everyone can implement into any lifestyle. Implementing a healthy diet, exercise for the brain, mind and body all combine to improve the state of our mental health. Defending ourselves from the thoughts that weaken and sicken our function of health by being virtuous. Choosing what is hearty for the mind, not our egos. Speaking in a compassionate and loving language towards ourselves and others.

Only together can we form the body of strength needed to change the world one person at a time. We might not be able to change the entire world, but we can change the entire world for that one person and that has a magically contagious effect. Each mind that opens has the potential to become healthy, mental illness or neurotypical alike. Most people give up their power by believing they do not have any. The media bolsters this point to control opinion and freedom of the mind. We can change this by sharing our strengths and weaknesses, showcasing how to take our power back and use it properly to help each other. Staying close to each other socially.

Most importantly we each need to become one drop of water. Become the one drop of water that creates a waterfall. Carve the way through the toughest of rock so that other drops of water will then be able to follow. We take a leap of faith when we fall into the unknown. When we look back, it will be full of happiness because together we all created an almighty waterfall. A harmonious and valuable contributor to a healthy and growing ecosystem that replenishes itself within its environment. Sustainable cycle through purpose making everything around it flourishes. An environment which is magnetic for positive attention in its dynamic simplicity. Providing new life with what is needed in which to survive. All created by one drop of water.

This is more paramount than ever given the current circumstances in our world today. We are programmed to think in big unattainable complex outcomes. Programmed to stay still. From my experience, simplifying and minimizing outcome and expectation made it very easy to think small. To shrink the unnecessary complexities within the strategy so that the battle plan becomes obvious and simply attainable.

Dreaming big is amazing, I'm just saying for me, thinking smaller makes everything unattainable become easily obtainable. Therefore, by simplifying the dream, I was able to manifest and then materialize my dream into reality by rewiring the programs within my mind and taking the obligatory action to trenches. Be one drop of water. Peaceful. Fluid. Purposeful.

Start your own waterfall. Share the magic of your story. Reconnect to the reconnection of social interaction with people. Express everything that we are by being genuine and vulnerable and people will follow our lead. Do it as soon as possible, as in right now. Every single person on this planet has a unique testament of their experiences that someone else will connect with and act based on that. We are all connected, and it is our responsibility to use that for powerful positive action. Conversations are everything. They are the reason we grow together, become closer, understand one and another, share and express creative ideas. The collective connections made inside our conversations are what shape our relationships and our contributions to them. Separation is not the answer, even though the psychological onslaught of propaganda on social media would want us to believe that it is, sadly it is working. We should be focusing on the possibilities and opportunities, not just pointing an opinionated finger at the problems. The answer to everything is epitomized in the solutions that we create to help make improvements and to make something better, not just for ourselves but for others we will never see it take place for. Always with the belief for the better good. It is up to the individual which way they choose to see unless self-induced ignorance has blinded that person temporarily. There is always hope when we choose to believe it. That belief is the inertia of the waterfall. Its driving force. One thought, one idea, one action is all it takes to start.

There is no perfect cure for mental illness. But there are antidotes. Antidotes are counteracting agents. From my experience these antidotes are all connected and associated within the environments we choose to live in. Physical activity, brain training, mental self-defense, embracing pain as a teacher, open mindedness, rewiring our brain, positive internal language, ego release and balancing, forgiveness, letting things be, meditation, virtuous thought command, self-disciple, self-respect and self-love through the transformation triangle, purpose, changing our habits, early mornings, honesty with ourselves, overcoming fear by comprehension and strategy planning, believing in what we can achieve, losing expectation and control, and learning that failure is not a bad thing at all. These are all antidotes for mental illness and help safeguard our mental health. Building a tolerance over time to the potency and toxicity of the venom. Healing old, infected wounds. Mending the parts of us that had come apart. Becoming healthy mentally and physically is the anti-venom. The harmonious cooperative alliance of exercise of the body, brain and the mind illustrate that no matter how turbulent the past was, becoming a peaceful warrior is possible in the present moment, when we stop repeating the suffering inflicted behavior patterns from our past. Allowing the opportunity to grow, to thrive, to illuminate and light the way through the darkness we once feared, incandescently diffusing away the shadows where the monster used to live.

JUNE 19, 2021

I know who I am,
The solace is flowing in my blood.
I can't be anything else.
Blind in light,
from the darkness
I no longer know how to see.
Hospital knives,
Don't need to fix me with surgery
Because I already saved,
the million beautiful people inside of me.
One last shiver,
Inside a chill
Looking into a mirror,
At the man, the monster cannot kill.

I had been sitting on the edge of my couch looking out the window off and on for about an hour. It was a warm, humid, and stormy summer morning. Dark bellied clouds blanketed the sky as far as I could see. It was raining out, pouring. I was watching the large raindrops fall from the sky in slow motion and then as they hit my window, watching the drops of water slither and snake their way down the glass eventually falling into a large puddle they were forming on my balcony. It was hypnotizing. Teardrops slid slowly down my face in synchronicity.

I was watching an intricately delicate ballet of cohesion and adhesion. A drop of water such as raindrop, teardrop or water drop are all held together by surface tension and all share the course of becoming too heavy and eventually falling from their host due to gravity, whether it be from condensation that gathers on a leaf in the forest and falls to the ground below it. A raindrop falling from an accumulation of vapor and rapid temperature change inside a Cumulonimbus Cloud. A teardrop created from the human eye.

The importance of water drops in our world are preeminent. Binding all life together by being its freshwater life source. Every body of water, big or small, carries an immense purpose in our ecosystems. Puddles, creeks, pools, swamps, marshes, ponds, streams, rivers, lakes, waterfalls, seas, and oceans all are dependent on the mighty raindrop for their existence. Rain being the proprietor, the giver of all life. Without rain and water vapor there would be no life on our planet. The rainfall on the oceans has a profound effect on our weather systems, climate, diluting salts through evaporation and temporarily altering the surface temperatures of the ocean. Obviously, an entire infinite orchestra of water drops are necessary to constantly renew these natural resources, which in turn provide life on land and in all bodies of water.

Every drop of water in a forest or jungle falls from the trees and leaves, landing on the richly organic layer of soils and debris below it. Thus, creating the opportunity for vegetation, fungi, aiding in decomposition of matter and providing plant and tree roots with a nourishing drink. The complex relationship of interaction with all the animals and plants that live there are unique to the biodiversity of its ecosystem, but all rely on water.

A teardrop may not have the significance of providing survival to living things. However, the teardrop has quite an implausible phenomenon unique to human beings. Many other animals have tear ducts just like we do, and their purpose is to provide a liquid to clean irritants from the eye. When dust, dirt, or smoke gets in the eye the tear duct will overflow with lubricant to wash away all irritants, cleansing the eye. A teardrop is composed primarily of water but also contains salt, fatty oils, electrolytes, vitamins, minerals and over fifteen hundred types of proteins.

We are the only animal alive that can generate teardrops through an emotional origin. We shed tears in response to a range of our feelings and emotions. These teardrops contain a higher level of stress hormones than other types. We cry at funerals, when relationships end, when we are saddened or hurt, suffering, but on the same note, we also cry at weddings, when a baby is born, we cry when we laugh uncontrollably, or when we hear or see someone triumph over life threatening odds we rejoice in happy tears. We often feel better after we cry and that is due to shedding emotional teardrops, releases endorphins and oxytocin within the brain. These chemicals make us humans feel good and can ease both emotional and physical pain. Quite the unique spectacle for our species indeed.

Outside my window, I looked at a tree that had been growing and blossoming. There were so many vibrant big green leaves decorated all over the mighty outreaching branches. The warm winds were from the south and gusting, rustling the leaves and the rain creating a beautiful natural symphony.

I had opened all the blinds on my windows and turned around into the brightness of my world. I wanted it as bright as possible. I wanted to see everything. I had so much more to see now. I recognized myself more than ever. I knew who I was. I was becoming who I was meant to be. I sat down on the floor beside my couch with my back against the wall. The tears I had were very heavy. Heavy with happiness. In fact, they were loaded with all the happiness I had ever felt in my life inside their composition.

Scattered all over the floor in front of me were letters, poems, and captured thoughts I had written down over the previous days and nights beforehand. I had been writing, exercising, learning, and growing. I had been eating healthy food and drinking so much water. Enhancing all the feelings of my memories of my family, friends and loved ones. It was time to finally put an end to the reign of terror from that monster which had controlled my mind since I was a little boy.

I was all alone. Running absolutely wild and free like an uncaged animal inside the fields, forests, and jungles in my head. Unconditional freedom. Untamed happiness. My thoughts were like bright colors that had impact, direction and full of life. My newfound freedom screamed, and it was the most attractive sound I had ever heard inside my mind. The only feeling I had was the release of happiness. My eyes were wide open, and I could see so many new colors for the very first time. Like paintings, everywhere that I looked.

I felt lighter and stronger than ever. Like a magnificent great hammerhead shark gliding weightlessly through the blue shimmer of a tropical ocean. Always moving forward, relentless in its process of fulfilling its purpose.

I told myself that the next teardrop that slid down my face and it fell to the floor, that I would begin my life. My mind had become an encouraging recollection of my time. It felt like an endless warm summer night. When it is still hot, but a breeze comes to calmly remind you that everything is just the way it should be. Tears began to form and roll down my face from my smiling eyes. They caressed my skin on their way. As one pause at the bottom of my jawline, gradually forming the shape of a teardrop, life as I knew it held flawlessly still. A moment where the whole entirety of my life was encapsulated within one tiny teardrop. All the experiences, memories and events that lead to all the perspective changing lessons that I was fortunate to have the opportunity to learn from, was all I felt. I could see all the people that I had helped, healed, loved, and made their hearts feel full of life. All the people I shared laughter with, created extraordinary memories with, had protected or lifted up, the ones who had been there for me when I needed it most. I could not feel any painful memories whatsoever. They had become checkpoints, references, and reminders of where I came from and where I was going. Every single moment of my life began flashing like a strobe light of snapshots. Like a slideshow. Speeding through so many of my memories. Some that I had no recollection of, and many that I did. From my birth to my childhood, my teenage years and then my adult life right up to the very moment in which I was living in. Reliving literally thousands of experiences at what felt like the speed of light, left my mind fluid and straightforward.

I was being serenaded by the echoes of all that I loved in my life and by the choir of boreal chorus frogs and spring peepers as I sat beside the still creek in my mind. Absolution cradled my hand as I picked the pen off the floor beside me. As I put the pen to the piece of paper, a powerful sensation that felt like warm sunlight on my face and throughout my body took over. For a brief second, I sat there, calm like a time bomb. Waiting. My mind was finally full for the first time that I could recall in my entire life. I had finally stopped running away. There I stood, face to face and smirked as I stared into the ravenous eyes of the monster that had been trying to kill me since I was a little boy.

As that teardrop liberated itself and fell from my face, suddenly time was released and no longer stood still. Reality hit like a bright flashing lightning strike as that one drop of water hit the floor. I took a last deep breath and closed my eyes, kissing the monster goodbye. I screamed as loud as I could silently inside my head.

Squeezing the pen,
I wrote these words.
Not today depression
Not today...

You are not alone. Please believe that. Even when all seems lost, there is a way back. It doesn't matter how far off the road you go; you won't get lost once you have found yourself, and sometimes that takes time. The feelings that are heavy and overwhelming will pass. The thoughts that are hurting you are temporary and can be altered. Depression is real. It has the potential to be a killer. I watched it seal my coffin. I know what it feels like to believe there is no other way out but to end it. To feel so alone and so meaningless that all hope is destroyed. Thinking the only way to stop feeling so bad everyday was to commit suicide. I was wrong. Very wrong. In fact, I have never been more wrong about anything in my life.

If you are having twisted thoughts and you cannot see any other way out, if you feel alone and that no one cares, and you are contemplating suicide. Please reconsider. This world needs you and is a better place because you are in it. There are people who care about you, and you are not meaningless. Hope will come back to you and guide you. There is help available for you. It will get better; it just takes some time. Every new day is a new chance for a new life. Someday, you will have the opportunity to share your story about how you conquered whatever it was that you went through, and it will become a survival guide for someone else that needs it. At the end of the day, if you cannot do it for someone you love, or stay alive for yourself, then please do it for me...

because I did this for you.

ABOUT THE AUTHOR

Jason Tyler McLean is a Winnipeg, Canada based author, speaker, and educator. He lives with mental illness and has made it his purpose to share his story to help empower others who are amid struggle with mental health issues, to influence in a positive way that through story telling and taking action that lives can transform, and improve the relationship with ourselves in hopes to establish better connection with each other. His vision is to unite as many minds as possible with the purpose of disabling the stigma that casts a dark shadow over mental health and mental illness.

He loves working out and anything fitness. Sharks, frogs, butterflies, and all other animals. Studying the brain, behavior, biology, and anything science related.

Travelling near and far, waterfalling, painting, plants, cycling, being in nature, and spending time with family, friends, and loved ones.

This is his first book...

Manufactured by Amazon.ca
Bolton, ON

29316747R00131